WHAT PEOPLE ARE SAYING ABOUT

Find and Follow Your Inner Compass

Following the simple approach in Barbara Berger's book – *Find and Follow Your Inner Compass* – can totally revolutionize your life. I know because it has revolutionized mine.
Tim Ray, author of *101 Relationship Myths* and the *Starbrow* Series

I recommend that everyone – no matter how difficult it may seem – follow Barbara Berger's book on the 'Inner Compass'. If I hadn't done so, I wouldn't be sitting here today, telling my story. Because understanding the 'Inner Compass' is the key to living a true and authentic life. Oh how easily we get off track. Thanks for everything, Barbara!
Jane Aamund, best-selling author of *Colorado Dreams*

Berger is a big name in the field of personal development with a large following. *Find and Follow Your Inner Compass* definitely lives up to her other books. The book is easy to read and use and every library should buy it and have it in stock.
The National Library

Everyone has an Inner Compass, but not everyone knows how to use it. Barbara Berger can help with this. In her beautiful new book, she guides you in how to experience a life with more flow and joy – by using your Inner Compass. And it's interesting reading indeed – because we all know about the dilemmas she describes. Strongly recommended!
The Family Guide

In her new book, Barbara Berger shows us how one can live a happy, abundant and fulfilling life in an increasingly turbulent world. According to Barbara Berger, the key is to pay attention to our feelings and live in harmony with who we really are. A simple recipe – not unlike what the Greek philosopher Epictetus said.

My Health

Find and Follow Your Inner Compass

Instant Guidance in an Age of Information Overload

Other books by Barbara Berger

The Road to Power
– Fast Food for the Soul

The Road to Power 2
– More Fast Food for the Soul

Gateway to Grace
– Barbara Berger's Guide to User-Friendly Meditation

Mental Technology (The 10 Mental Laws)
– Software for Your Hardware

The Spiritual Pathway
– A Guide to the Joys of Awakening and Soul Evolution

The Adventures of Pebble Beach

Are You Happy Now?
10 Ways to Live a Happy Life

The Awakening Human Being
– A Guide to the Power of Mind (with Tim Ray)

Sane Self Talk
– Cultivating the Voice of Sanity Within

Find and Follow Your Inner Compass

Instant Guidance in an Age of Information Overload

Barbara Berger

BOOKS

Winchester, UK
Washington, USA

First published by O-Books, 2017
O-Books is an imprint of John Hunt Publishing Ltd., Laurel House, Station Approach,
Alresford, Hants, SO24 9JH, UK
office1@jhpbooks.net
www.johnhuntpublishing.com

For distributor details and how to order please visit the 'Ordering' section on our website.

Text copyright: Barbara Berger 2016

ISBN: 978 1 78099 510 6
978 1 78099 512 0 (ebook)
Library of Congress Control Number: 2016949321

A CIP catalogue record for this book is available from the British Library.

Design: Stuart Davies

Cover photo: Søren Solkaer

Printed and bound by CPI Group (UK) Ltd, Croydon, CR0 4YY, UK

We operate a distinctive and ethical publishing philosophy in all
areas of our business, from our global network of authors to
production and worldwide distribution.

CONTENTS

Foreword

Thanks to the great advances in technology and the wonders of social media, never before in human history have we human beings been so plugged into each other. Never before have we had constant online access to what everyone else is thinking, saying, feeling and doing.

So in this time, when we are bombarded from morning to evening with information from all sides as to what is best and what we "should" and "shouldn't" do to live happy lives, how can anyone navigate through this massive sea of information and know what's best for them to do in any given situation? In other words, is there a reliable way to make decisions and navigate wisely through life? Is there a way that takes into consideration who each individual is and what his or her needs, wants and desires are?

And the answer to this question is yes, there is a way!

Because every single person alive has an Inner Compass! Every person has his or her own unique, personal, internal guidance system – which is working at all times and which is each individual's direct connection to the Great Universal Intelligence that created each one of us and all of Life.

And that's what this book is all about. It's about how to find, understand and use your internal guidance system – which I call the "Inner Compass" – to live a happier, more fulfilling, exciting and wonderful life.

This book is based on the understanding that – not only do you have an Inner Compass, but that your Inner Compass is, in each and every moment, giving you precise and reliable information as to what is the best way forward for you in every situation in your life. And how does the Inner Compass do this? It does so by means of your emotions. That is why I explore and explain the true significance of our emotions in this book and describe, in detail, how and why our emotions are important and significant indicators of whether or not we are in alignment with who we really are and the Great Universal Intelligence that has created all of us.

So I hope that, as you read, consider, digest and absorb the information presented here, it will help you learn to listen to and follow your Inner Compass on a daily basis. And that as a result, you will be able to live more fully in alignment with who you truly are and what is uniquely suitable for you (and not for anyone else). When this happens, you will experience more flow, ease, joy, love, passion and enthusiasm in your life – and as a result experience the joy of being of greater service to your family, friends, colleagues, and to the world in general.

To make it easier for you to digest and absorb the information presented here about the Inner Compass, I have divided this book into two sections.

In Part One, I cover the basics: What is the Inner Compass and how does it work? How do we read the signals the Inner Compass is giving us in every now moment? What is the true significance of our emotions? How do we use the Inner Compass in practice – in our everyday lives, at work, in our relationships?

In Part Two, I address the challenges that arise such as: What sabotages our ability to listen to and follow our Inner Compass? Is it selfish to follow the Inner Compass – what about the other people in our lives? How can we constructively deal with the fear of other people's disapproval, especially when the Inner Compass points us in a direction we believe other people will disapprove of or dislike? How can we gradually improve our ability to listen to and follow our Inner Compass?

Throughout the book, there are also concrete examples of using the Inner Compass in our daily lives.

The information presented in this book is based on many years of private sessions coaching people and seeing the amazing transformations that occur in people's lives when they start understanding and applying the principles in this book. That is how I know embracing the Inner Compass can work for you – because I've seen it work for so many other people, regardless of their age, gender, financial status, health conditions, relation- ships or any other circumstances. No matter who you are or where you are in your life, the Inner Compass can and is working for you!

May this book help you live the full, rich, exciting life you were born to live!

Good reading!

Barbara Berger
Copenhagen
December 2015

PART ONE:

You have an Inner Compass

You have an Inner Compass

You have an Inner Compass. You have an amazingly accurate and reliable Inner Compass that is working all the time. An Inner Compass that is constantly giving you guidance and information as to what is best for you and whether or not you are in alignment with who you really are.

And how does the Inner Compass do this? It does this by means of your emotions. Your emotions are the way in which the Inner Compass lets you know how you are doing. When you feel good, when you feel a sense of ease and flow, enthusiasm and joy in your life, these good-feeling emotions are an indication that you are in alignment with who you really are. When you feel less than good, when you feel a sense of discomfort, frustration, overwhelmed, anxious or distressed in any way, these negative emotions are an indication that you are out of alignment and not doing what's best for you.

So the Inner Compass is a very simple mechanism. It is an internal yes/no mechanism that is your direct connection to the Great Universal Intelligence – that Greater Intelligence that created this amazing Universe and all Life in it, including you. In order to provide you with a clear indication of whether or not you are in alignment with what the Greater Intelligence knows to be the truth about you, the Inner Compass works like the North/South guidance of an ordinary directional compass. When you are in alignment – when you are living in harmony with who you really are and what is best for you – this Inner Compass points directly North and you feel a sense of comfort, ease and flow in your life. In other words, you feel good. And when you're not in alignment with who you really are (with the North/South position), it means you are off the beam, and as a result, you feel a sense of discomfort or unease. In other words, you don't feel so good.

It's as simple as that.

But unfortunately, most people have lost touch with their Inner Compass, which is their very own, natural internal guidance system. As a result, most of us don't realize that this is what our emotions are all about. We don't understand or realize that our emotions are actually indicators, which are all the time telling us whether or not we are in alignment with who we really are and with what is best for us, in any and every given moment in time or situation.

So the heart of the matter is that your emotions matter! How you feel matters!

Everyone knows when something feels good or bad, everyone knows the difference between feeling angry and feeling love, between feeling depressed and feeling joyful... but what most of us don't understand or realize is that these emotions are important indicators because they are giving us vital information about what is going on in our lives. So when you stop and notice what's going on inside you, you will see you are probably experiencing a wide range of emotions, emotions which vary, depending on the situation you are in. Whether it's what's going on in your family or what's happening as you interact with your partner or your colleagues at work.

But whether we are aware of this mechanism or not, our emotions are there! All the time. And this means that, whether we know it or not, each one of us has an Inner Compass that is providing us with this information by means of our emotions. So when you start to notice, you will see that this Inner Compass is always telling you in each and every moment in time – how you feel about what is going on in your life. Your emotions are giving you this valuable information all of the time. And this internal guidance system is always on, always available, always giving you second by second, minute by minute information and guidance, which you can use to make wise choices for yourself in every situation.

But unfortunately most people don't know about the Inner Compass and don't know that our emotions are the key to understanding and using this internal guidance system.

Understanding our emotions

Since our emotions are the key to understanding how our Inner Compass works, let's take a look at them. We human beings have many words to describe the different states or emotions that we experience, but we can categorize all our emotions under two basic categories or emotional states – *Comfort* and *Discomfort*. All our emotions fit into one of these categories. Here are some examples of how our emotions fit into these 2 categories:

Comfort	Discomfort
Love	Fear
Happiness	Depression
Joy	Anxiety
Ease	Unease
Excitement	Stress
Passion	Anger
Flow	Resistance
Enthusiasm	Irritation
Satisfaction	Grouchy
Peace	Agitation
Fun	Boredom
Harmony	Disharmony
Etc.	Etc.
In other words, good-feeling emotions	In other words, not good-feeling emotions

The good-feeling emotions give a sense of ease and flow, while the not-good-feeling emotions give a sense of unease, discomfort and resistance.

And this is what the Inner Compass is telling you. This is the information the Inner Compass is giving you all the time. By means of your emotions, the Inner Compass is giving you a direct and precise readout as to what you are feeling in every moment. And these feelings are the way in which your Inner Compass tells you whether you are in alignment or not, in terms of who you are and what is going on right now. So all you have to notice, or ask yourself, is this: How does it feel? How does this situation feel? How does this person feel? How does this thought feel? Am I feeling a sense of comfort/ease/flow or a sense of discomfort/unease/resistance about this person, situation, circumstance – or even about myself?

In this connection, it is important to understand that your Inner Compass is not telling you whether things are so-called "right" or "wrong" or "correct" or "incorrect". It is only telling you how you really "feel", in terms of whatever is going on in relation to who you really are – and it's telling you about what's happening right this very moment.

So when you and what you are thinking and doing are in alignment with who you really are and what's best for you, you are in harmony with who you really are. Which translates into a feeling of joy, flow, ease and happiness because you are living in alignment with your true nature, your deeper essence, or you could say with your soul essence. And then, the connection is open between you and the Great Universal Intelligence that is orchestrating the dance of Life. So Life feels good and is good and you are in flow – and things just seem to work out better for you.

I know it sounds very simple – and it is.

The simple truth is we feel better when we are living in alignment with who we really are and are allowing the flow of Life to stream through us – fully and freely – so that each one of us can live out our own unique destiny path.

How do I know that everyone has an Inner Compass?

The Great Universal Intelligence

To answer this question, let's start by taking a look at what's really going on. Let's take a look at the world, at reality. Did you notice that the sun came up this morning? Well, yes, you say, it did. The sun did come up this morning. And I say, so may I ask – did you make the sun come up this morning? Did you do it? Did you make the sun come up? Was it on your "to do" list or did the sun just come up by itself? And you answer, no, you didn't make the sun come up this morning. It came up without your help. And then I ask, what about the planets orbiting in space – are you making that happen? No, you say again, it isn't you. And what about the trees growing outside and the grass and the plants, I continue. Are you making all that happen? Again, you answer no. And what about the seas and the oceans and all the fish and all the other animals? Are you making any of them happen? No, you answer again, you are not. But something is happening, we can all see that. We can all see that the sun does come up every morning and that the planets are revolving around the sun in perfect harmony every day and that the plants are arising and growing and the animals are there – and that all this is happening and we are not making it happen. We are not doing it. Not you and not me. But it is happening anyway, I say.

So from this, we can conclude that there is some Force or Greater Intelligence that is creating, manifesting and organizing this amazing Web of Life, this amazing dance which is our Cosmos. There is some Greater Intelligence or Force which is creating and orchestrating all of this – and this is what I mean when I say the Great Universal Intelligence. I mean this greater creative Force or Power or Intelligence (or whatever else you might want to call it) that is organizing and coordinating the unfolding of Life all around us.

Something is there and something is doing all of this. It's obvious. You can see it unfolding wherever you look.

We can also ask the same questions when we look at

11

ourselves. So let's try that.

If you take a look at yourself, I can ask you – did you create your own body? Did you make yourself appear in this body? And again, you answer no. You did not make you happen, but again, here you are! You are here in this body, right here, right now. So something greater, some greater intelligence, which is far more intelligent than you or I, has organized and animated and manifested YOU!

The other thing about you (and me) is that now that we're here, we're still not "doing" us. By this I mean, you are not making yourself "be", you are just happening! Just think about it. Do you sit up all night and tell your heart to beat? No, you don't. Yet your heart beats all night long all by itself, without you telling it what to do, or watching it, or doing anything. It just does. Your heart just beats. And the same goes for your lungs, which continue to breathe the air in and out, in and out. And the same with your digestion, which keeps on digesting your food and all the other millions and trillions of cells and processes in your body, which are all going on all by themselves – without any thought, or direction, or interference from you or me. So again, there is some greater intelligence at work here. There must be some Force or Intelligence that has manifested you and me and everyone else and which is now animating and coordinating these amazing physical bodies, which we all have.

Just think about the intelligence of our bodies!

If, for example, you cut your finger with a knife while you are out in the kitchen preparing lunch and your finger starts to bleed… what do you do? Probably you will wash your finger off and then put a bandage on it. And once your finger is all bandaged up, you will probably just forget all about it. You'll just forget it and leave it alone. Then a couple of days later, you'll take off the bandage and see what you knew would happen – the cut has grown back together. All by itself, just as you knew it would. And it all happened by itself, so to speak. It all happened automatically. It just did.

You didn't sit there looking at your finger, all day long and all night long, telling the cells of your body to grow back together. The cells in your body knew what do to and they did it automatically – without any direction from you or interference from you. So who or what was doing it? Again, there is, obviously, some Greater Intelligence at work here. Obviously!

So this is what I mean by the Great Universal Intelligence. I mean that Greater Intelligence or organizing power that has created and manifested all of creation including you and me!

And now we come to what I call the Inner Compass. Since this Great Universal Intelligence created you and is animating you, it must be *in you*. And this is what I mean by the Inner Compass. The Inner Compass is your connection to and awareness of the Great Universal Intelligence.

The Inner Compass is the Great Universal Intelligence manifesting itself in you! And this is why it's so important to understand and use your Inner Compass – because it's your direct link, your direct connection, to the Great Universal Intelligence, which is that All-Powerful Infinite Energy that has created and is animating all of Life – all of this entire, amazing, wondrous Infinite Universe – including you. And this Life Force, which is All-Powerful, All-Knowing Infinite Energy and Infinite Intelligence, is also Infinite Aliveness. And when we experience this Infinite Aliveness, it feels like joy and it feels like love and it feels like passion and enthusiasm and appreciation.

So when you feel like this – when you feel good, when you feel a sense of well-being – you know that you are in harmony with the great flow of Life that is manifesting through you. In other words, you are in harmony with the Great Universal Intelligence that is flowing through you. When this happens, you feel so amazing, you feel so good, you feel so happy! And this is why your emotions matter! This is why your emotions are significant. Because they are telling you where you are in relation to the real you – in relation to the real you that is living in harmony with the great flow of Life. So the better you feel, the better something feels, the more in harmony with Life and the Great Universal Intelligence you are! In fact, the good-feeling emotions are the way in which the Great Universal Intelligence is saying to you – loud and clear – *You're on the right track... you are on the right track... so go for it! GO FOR IT!*

Not in contact with the Inner Compass

The shocking truth, however, is that many of us have lost contact with our Inner Compass – with our connection to this Great Universal Intelligence – and so we have lost contact with our own internal guidance system. And because of this, we are not truly in contact with how we really feel about things and so we flounder in our life situations and life becomes a struggle. I know this sounds strange, but it is true nevertheless.

So how can this be?

There are two main reasons why so many people are not in contact with their Inner Compass. Firstly: Ignorance or lack of awareness of the Inner Compass! Simply put, we don't know the Inner Compass exists. We don't know we have an Inner Compass because no one ever told us about it. So we never learned that we have an Inner Compass. Our parents didn't teach us about it because they didn't know about it either. And they didn't know about it because their parents didn't teach them about the Inner Compass either! And so it goes, back through the generations. Not that many people have ever been aware of this mechanism, and as a result, information about this mechanism has not been readily available before. And because of this, we didn't know about the Inner Compass and we don't teach our children about the Inner Compass either.

Just think about it. Can you remember anyone ever saying to you in your childhood that you have an Inner Compass – an internal guidance system – that you can depend upon and that is always telling you what is best for you in any given situation? Did anyone ever tell you about this? Did anyone ever tell you that this was what your emotions were all about? That your emotions were important and that they were signals? That your emotions were the way in which your Inner Compass – your internal guidance system – was conveying this information to you? Can you remember anyone ever saying anything like that? Did your parents ever explain to you that only you could know what's best for you because you are the only one who's inside you and the only one who has access to your Inner Compass? Did they tell you that you were the only one who knows how things feel to you? Did they tell you that you were the only person in the whole wide Universe who has contact with your internal guidance system? Did your teachers tell you this? Or your friends? Did anyone, in fact, ever tell you about this mechanism?

Probably not.

And I can say this with some certainty because I've been coaching and counseling people all my life and so far I've never met anyone who could honestly answer yes to this question. Who could honestly say that they know they have an internal guidance system because their parents taught them this in their childhood. So the reality is, most of us don't even know that this Inner Compass exists. We simply don't know that we have an internal guidance system that is always with us and is always working.

And then there's the second reason.

In addition to the fact that we don't know we have an Inner Compass that can guide and direct us in every aspect of our daily lives, most of us have been trained (programmed and indoctrinated) from early childhood to make most of our decisions and to say and do things mainly to please other people. We have been trained like this because we learned at an early age that if we wanted things to go well for us, it was a good idea to please the grown-ups around us. That's the way we were brought up. That's the way we were programmed. The messages we got in early childhood were usually very clear and told us in no uncertain terms – *it's important to please other people.* It's important that other people approve of you and what you are saying and doing. So we learned at an early age that things would go better for us if we pleased the people around us. We got the message from our parents, in a million ways, that said, "Things will go better for you if you do what I want you to do." Or "I'll love you if you do what I want."

So from an early age, we were trained to notice and pay attention, all of the time, to what we believed (or learned to believe) other people were and are expecting from us so that we can make them happy. We got the message, early on, that it's our job to make other people happy. So we've been trained to have our antennas out, trained to focus on other people, instead of turning inward and focusing on the information that is coming from our internal guidance system, which is inside of us.

You were probably taught that your feelings didn't really matter

So basically what happened is we learned from an early age that our feelings don't matter. Since no one understood the true significance of emotions, we were taught from childhood to disregard our feelings. In other words, it was okay to feel bad as long as you pleased other people. So we learned from early on not to pay too much attention to what is going on inside of us and instead to notice, be aware of, and fall in line with what the people around us were expecting of us.

Please let me be clear here – I am not talking about allowing children to become spoiled brats and creating families with no healthy boundaries and no basic house rules or clear guidelines for respectful behavior between people. (For more about this, see The Inner Compass and children on page 78.) What I am talking about here is our basic misunderstandings about this thing called Life, which includes the fact that people are different, with different ideas and agendas (even in the same family), and that each person has his or her own direct link to the Great Universal Intelligence, which created us all and which is providing each one of us with information about who we are and what is in alignment with each of us and our life path.

So even if most of us will say that we know what feels good and what feels bad, that's not the point here. The point is the significance of how we feel. The point is that our emotions are indicators, which are providing us with important – yes vital – information about our own alignment with who we really are. This is what is so important to understand. That good feelings are a signal from within, a signal from your Inner Compass, that you are living in alignment with who you really are. And negative emotions are also a signal from within that you are out of alignment or off course... So it's important to understand that your emotions are a reliable source of information and guidance, regardless of what other people are saying.

So you can see... it's all been rather backwards for most of us, right from the beginning.

And as a result of this, most of us don't understand what our emotions mean and have lost contact with our Inner Compass.

So the big question is – how do we get in contact with our Inner Compass again?

To answer this question, I have designed the following exercise to help you find and follow your Inner Compass again. And here it is:

The Inner Compass exercise – here's what to do:

The Inner Compass exercise is all about finding and using your Inner Compass every day in every situation. This is what you do.

First of all, start thinking about and contemplating the fact that you have an Inner Compass. Read the first pages of this book over and over again until you really "get" it. Then make the decision that you are going to be mindful of the fact that you have an Inner Compass during the course of your day. That you are going to remember, and remind yourself, that you have an Inner Compass. Then start noticing how you feel, really feel, at various times during the course of your day.

Notice when things feel good and notice when they don't.

Notice when you feel good and when you don't.

And then – again during the course of your day – when you notice that you are thinking more about what other people may be thinking or feeling about you – or about a situation, event, or another person – than what you yourself are thinking and feeling, immediately pull back your focus from the other people and return your focus to yourself. In other words, when you catch yourself worrying about what your boss is thinking, or about what your partner is thinking, or about what your mother is thinking, just drop it.

Drop the thought of what anyone else might be thinking or feeling about what's going on. Drop it like you've got a hot potato in your hand and it's burning you! Ouch! That hurts, so drop it. Drop the hot potato! Drop trying to figure out what other people may or may not be thinking or feeling or wanting. Just let it go. Just drop trying to figure out what anyone else is thinking and feeling about what's going on and gently return to yourself.

Then take a deep breath and go within and *notice what you are feeling*. In other words, notice what your Inner Compass is telling you about the present situation, or about the person you are confronted with, or about whatever is going on before you right now.

In other words, take a moment to go within and just notice how *this* feels to you right now. How does *this* situation feel? How does *this* person feel? How does *this* event feel right now?

That's what the Inner Compass is telling you. And that's what the Inner Compass exercise is all about.

It's about noticing.

It's about noticing honestly.

It's about present-moment awareness.

It's about right now.

It's about being mindful of what's going on within you, right this moment.

It's about being mindful of your own unique connection to the Great Universal Intelligence.

It's about being mindful of the fact that you have an Inner Compass that is always giving you direct, real-time information as to how things feel and what is best for you.

It's about understanding what your emotions mean and that they matter.

This is what the Inner Compass is all about and this is what the Inner Compass is telling you. It's telling you how things feel to you right now. So ask yourself: How does this feel right now? Does this situation, event or person feel good or not? Does this give you a sense of comfort or discomfort? That's all you have to notice.

Just notice.

Notice how you actually feel.

And then keep doing this. Make it your daily practice to notice, every day, as often as you can during the course of your day, how things are feeling to you. In other words, notice what your Inner Compass is telling you. Does this situation or person give you a sense of comfort or discomfort? How does it make you feel? Does it feel good or not? That's all you have to do.

Just notice your Inner Compass and listen to what it's telling you.

That's all there is to it.

It sounds simple, doesn't it?

But as simple as this may sound, this is not an easy thing for most people to do, especially in the beginning. And this is because we have been trained to, and have become so used to, focusing on other people and on trying to please other people. Most of us have learned from an early age to try to tune ourselves into what other people are wanting and needing. And as I said above, because of this we have lost contact with ourselves. We have lost contact with our Inner Compass and don't know how to tune into it anymore. So in the beginning, when using this exercise, it will feel rather strange, because we have become so used to focusing our attention away from ourselves. It will feel odd to stop focusing on other people and turn our attention back to ourselves.

But this is what using your Inner Compass is all about: Turning your attention away from other people and focusing on yourself.

So just keep reminding yourself of what this is all about. Then return to the Inner Compass over and over again. Be mindful when you realize that once again you are focusing on other people and worrying about what they might be thinking, saying or doing – and not listening to your internal guidance system. And don't beat up on yourself when you discover that you are doing this. Just understand that this is the way you've been trained and that now you are trying to learn a new, more appropriate, healthier way of being in the world.

So when you discover you've lost contact with yourself or are losing contact with yourself and are focusing solely on others and worrying about what they are thinking – just withdraw your attention from them and return home to yourself. The same goes for when you notice you're worrying about what one particular person (like your mother or your partner) may be thinking or believing about whatever is going on. Whoever it is – whether it's people in general or someone in particular – when you notice you are doing this, just gently withdraw your attention from the other person or people and return your attention to yourself.

And ask yourself – what does my Inner Compass say about this? Then just notice what comes up. Do you feel a sense of ease and flow about the present situation or person, or do you feel discomfort and resistance? That's all you're supposed to do.

Just notice.

So to summarize the exercise, here are the main steps:

The Inner Compass Exercise:

1) Think about and contemplate the fact that you have an Inner Compass. Reread this book, especially the first pages.

2) Make the decision to be mindful of your Inner Compass during the course of your day.

3) Start noticing how you feel at various times during the day and remember that your emotions matter.

4) When you notice that you are thinking about or worrying about what other people may be thinking – drop it.

5) Return to yourself and notice how you are feeling instead. Pay attention to your emotions.

Check in regularly with your Inner Compass

If you are new to noticing and following your Inner Compass in a more conscious way, it can be helpful to make it a habit to check in and notice your Inner Compass at various times during the course of your day. Again, just stop briefly and notice what kind of impulses your Inner Compass is giving you right this moment. Ask yourself – what feels good to me right now? In what direction do I feel the most ease and flow? Does it feel better to work on this project – or to take a break and work on something else? Does it feel good to make that phone call or not? And what about tonight? Do I really want to go to the movies with my friends? Or does it feel better to have some quiet time at home? And what about that invitation to that dinner party next weekend – how does that feel? What is the Inner Compass saying? And the situation at work – the one that has arisen between some of the team members. Does it feel good to call for a meeting and say something to the team? Or does it feel better to just let it be for the moment?

So again, during the course of your day ask yourself – what feels best to me right now, in this very moment, in this particular situation? And then just notice how you feel.

You already are following your Inner Compass in a lot of ways!

When you start working with the Inner Compass, you'll probably notice that you already are following your Inner Compass in lots of ways... you just haven't really noticed it before. At least not consciously. But yes, you are. Because instinctively, we are all being pulled towards what feels best. Just think about it. You know what you like best for breakfast – whether it's cereal or oatmeal or eggs and toast. Whether it's coffee or tea. You know what kind of jobs you're attracted to and what jobs would simply bore you to death. And the same goes for books and movies. You know what kind of stories excite you and what doesn't. And when it comes to going on holiday, you also know that. Maybe you love the mountains. Or maybe you prefer the big city. Or a tropical paradise. You are always being drawn towards the kind of places that feel good to you. And the same goes for music – you know what makes your heart sing and what doesn't... So you see, you are already following your Inner Compass in lots of ways, a lot of the time, without even noticing – quite simply, because it is natural for each one of us to be drawn to what makes us feel good. Everyone is naturally drawn toward what makes them feel more in the flow of Life because that is what feels best and most natural.

So the reality is, it feels good to be in harmony with who you really are and do what feels good! And this is true for everyone! Everyone likes to feel good.

Then of course, you will probably notice there are some areas in your life where you are actually going against the signals from your Inner Compass. Areas where you are forcing yourself to do things that don't feel good to you. When you notice this, you will probably also discover that you're doing what doesn't feel good either because you think you "should" or because you fear what other people might think of you if you don't do it!

Now, isn't that interesting?

Afraid to notice how you feel?

Here's another thing I've discovered when working with people. In the beginning, some people are almost afraid to do the Inner Compass exercise because they think that if they really HONESTLY notice how they feel about something, they will have to act immediately in accordance with this information. So I always say to people in the beginning: "Just start by doing the exercise to just notice how you truly feel. You don't have to take action on what you discover in the beginning. Just do the exercise and see what comes up."

I say this because I've discovered it might be too stressful or anxiety-provoking for some people, especially if they have been real people pleasers most of their lives, to suddenly find out that their Inner Compass is telling them something quite different from what they've been doing most of the time!

So when you start working with your Inner Compass, I suggest you be kind to yourself and start slowly. Just start by noticing how you actually feel at different times during your day, and in different situations. Just relax and notice what your Inner Compass is saying. Just observe. Because your Inner Compass is always there, is always providing you with accurate information about how things actually feel in relation to who you really are and what's most in harmony with you. So just try to relax and notice this.

That's all you have to do to begin with.

Just notice how you feel and try to be as HONEST as you can about it. In other words, try to be honest with yourself when you notice what's going on inside you, without worrying about the consequences of what you are discovering. Just let yourself feel how you really feel.

Change starts happening naturally and automatically

Then, as you start to get used to noticing your Inner Compass and the information it is giving you, you will find yourself naturally making small adjustments and changes in your life. This just happens automatically. Not so much because you "should" or because you "have to" but because it feels natural and good to do so. As you begin listening more consciously to your Inner Compass, you will find that making adjustments just feels good and actually resonates with who you really are. So this is not something you need to force, it is just something that will unfold naturally and happen automatically as you begin to feel more comfortable trusting your Inner Compass and being you.

Maybe you will find yourself taking the day off from work just because you feel like you need some time off. And while you are lying on your sofa, allowing yourself to recharge your batteries a little, you suddenly remember how you used to love to paint when you were younger. And lo' and behold, next time you are in town, your Inner Compass lets you know it feels good to stop at the artist supplies shop and buy some paint and paper... and then... and then...

You never know what you might discover when you start listening to those signals from within!

Your Inner Compass is not mental

Since your Inner Compass is all about feeling, we can deduce that the Inner Compass is not a mental thing. It's not about thinking things through or rationalizing things or explaining things. Your Inner Compass only tells you one thing – whether it feels good or not. In other words, whether you are in alignment with you and the Great Universal Intelligence or not. That's what the Inner Compass is doing – and it is giving you this information by means of your feelings.

So, as I said, your job is to notice how you feel about whatever is going on. Does it feel good or not? If the answer is yes, it feels good, then you are in alignment with who you really are. And this is not something you can think yourself to (quite simply because there are too many factors involved for our limited, rational minds to grasp). And this is why the Inner Compass is a feeling thing, a feeling barometer. So the only question you need to ask is – how does this feel? Does it give you a sense of comfort or discomfort? That's the information you are supposed to notice right now. And if it feels good, then it is good for you, right now. And only for right now.

I know this sounds amazingly simple to most of us because we're so used to trying to figure things out – to think our way to answers. But the tricky part about trying to figure things out and think our way to solutions is that in every single moment in time, there are always so many different factors involved. In fact, there is always an infinity of factors and aspects involved in every single situation. So not only is it impossible to figure everything out, but by trying to think our way to the so-called "best" solution – we tend to overlook our emotions. We tend to overlook how we actually feel about whatever is going on.

This is why the Inner Compass is such an interesting and vital mechanism – because it's based on the importance of our feelings, which most of us have misunderstood and overlooked.

So the basic premise is – *if something feels good to you then it is good for you.* And that's a pretty amazing concept for most of us because we have been trained away from trusting our own natural instincts and feelings, and our own inner guidance, into believing that we have to do all kinds of stuff that doesn't feel good to us in order to please other people.

The Inner Compass and the Great Universal Intelligence

So if our Inner Compass isn't mental, then what is it? How does it know what it knows? As I said at the beginning of this book, there is a Greater Intelligence, which I call the Great Universal Intelligence, that is creating, organizing and choreographing everything in creation – from the smallest to the greatest, at every moment in time. An intelligence that is so vast and so far beyond human comprehension. And our Inner Compass is our direct link or connection to this Great Universal Intelligence – to this greater knowingness. But it is important to understand that our limited, human, rational minds (with their logical and sequential way of thinking and analyzing) cannot grasp or understand this greater knowingness. Our minds are simply incapable of processing and understanding and/or comprehending everything that's going on in this amazing Infinite Universe at any given moment in time. The amount of information is just too vast and too fast changing. But the Great Universal Intelligence, the cosmic computer, which is beyond the comprehension of our logical minds, can and is doing this. And this is why when we listen to the signals from our Inner Compass (which is our connection to the Great Universal Intelligence), we are guided and directed beyond our own logical ability to "think" our way to the same conclusions.

And remember – the way the Great Universal Intelligence is giving us this information is via our emotions, which are giving us an instantaneous readout on our relationship to what's going on, which is, in fact, the whole of creation!

Thus, the Great Universal Intelligence – which simultaneously synchronizes everything in the whole Universe from the flocks of birds flying south overhead to the shoals of fishes in the great oceans swimming together as one mind, to the perfect dance of the planets revolving around the sun, and the vast galaxies swirling in space – is also providing you with perfect guidance if you will but listen in. Therefore, when you follow your Inner Compass, not only are you doing what is best for you – you are also doing what's best for the whole. Even if it is beyond the ability of your rational mind (or anyone else's) to understand this or explain why! This is also why the Wise Ones say, "The Good of One is the Good of All"!

Is it selfish to listen to your Inner Compass?

When I coach people to find and follow their Inner Compass, they often ask, "But isn't it selfish to follow my Inner Compass?" This question comes from an honest place because almost everyone I work with has high integrity and wants to be of benefit to the world and help other people. And this, of course, is a good thing. We all want to contribute to the welfare of the world and be of support to the people in our lives – which is another way of saying – we all want to love and be loving.

So here's my answer. First of all, it is important to understand that if you feel lousy, or ill, or depressed, or are stressed out of your mind, it's going to be very hard for you to function in your own life. Which also makes it very difficult for you to be of benefit to other people. I sometimes work with people who are on sick leave because of stress and when we go into their stories, it's obvious that they finally collapsed because of their own inability to say "no", set limits, and take good care of themselves. In other words, they were not following their Inner Compass. As a result, they ended up stressed out and ill. Which unfortunately greatly reduced their ability to be of benefit to the people in their lives (which was what they wanted to do in the first place).

So from this point of view, it's pretty obvious that listening to your Inner Compass makes sense if you want to be of benefit to the world. And this is whether we are talking about being a good parent or partner at home, or a good boss or colleague at work. Taking good care of yourself is a prerequisite to taking good care of others, no matter where you are and what you do. So it's important to take good enough care of yourself so you can feel good and be supportive of those around you.

It's a little like flying in an airplane with small children. I have three sons so I remember how it was when I flew with them when they were little. The stewardess explained that if the pressure in the cabin dropped and the oxygen masks came down over our heads, it was important for me (the mother) to put my own mask on first – before I helped my children. This is because if a mother puts the masks on her children first and then drops dead from lack of oxygen – how can she help them? So we're talking about the same principle here. *Help yourself first, so you can help others. Take good care of yourself first, so you can take good care of others.*

But there's another important aspect to all this too. When we say "being selfish" – what exactly do we mean by the "self" we are being selfish about? Are we talking about the little "self" – the ego or personality, which says "me, me, me", or are we talking about our connection to our True Selves which is what the Inner Compass is all about. Because if we are talking about our True Selves, then listening to the Inner Compass cannot possibly be "selfish" in the small sense of the word. Because the Inner Compass is our connection to the Great Universal Intelligence which knows our True Selves and which takes everything (and everyone) into consideration and is orchestrating the whole, vast and amazing dance of this entire infinite Universe. And if that is the case, which it is, then by tuning into this Greater Intelligence, we are aligning ourselves with the Wisdom of the Whole, which is always moving towards greater and greater balance and harmony... which translates for us into more Good, more Love, more Generosity for ourselves and the whole world... which,

again, is why it's such a good idea to listen to your Inner
Compass.

The Emotional Scale and keeping your energy high

In this connection, there's another interesting aspect to taking
good care of yourself. When I say taking good care of yourself –
I mean being in alignment with your True Self and the Great
Universal Intelligence. Because when this happens – when you
are in alignment – you feel good and your energy is high. Now
why is taking good care of yourself and keeping your energy
high so important when it comes to being a positive influence in
the world and helping other people?

To answer this question, let's look at the Emotional Scale
below, which shows the different emotions and the different
levels of energy and frequencies of these emotions. Because this
is another good way of looking at and understanding the information the Inner Compass is giving you.

Everyone knows there are good-feeling emotions and not so
good-feeling emotions. One can also say that the good-feeling
emotions and the not so good-feeling emotions represent
different levels of energy. And by different levels of energy, I
mean the different frequencies the energies are vibrating at.
Because the way the different energies actually "feel" tells us
what frequency an emotion is vibrating on. Because the different
emotions or feelings vibrate at different frequencies.

Just think about your emotions… and you know immediately
that they feel differently. Everyone can feel the difference
between feeling angry and feeling love. Everyone can feel the
difference between feeling depressed and feeling happy. Or the
difference between being confused and being clear. We all know
that these are quite different and distinct feelings. And the energy
of these different emotions feels quite different and distinct as
well.

We all also know that the energies of depression, fear or

anxiety make us feel heavy, lonely, and make us want to withdraw from life. While the energies of love, passion and enthusiasm make us feel open, and happy, and make us feel excited about life.

So that's what I mean when I say the various emotions or feelings are vibrating at different frequencies. And these frequencies make us feel in different ways. And as we have discovered, some emotions or energies make us feel good, while others make us feel less good about ourselves and life.

On a scale from high to low, the more good feeling an emotion is, the higher the vibrational frequency. The less good feeling an emotion is, the lower the vibrational frequency.

So if we categorize our feelings/emotions on an emotional scale from the lower to the higher frequencies, we will get a list that looks like this on a scale from lower (at the bottom of the list, opposite) to higher at the top:

The Emotional Scale

High, good-feeling energy
Love / Unconditional Love / Peace / Appreciation / Passion
Mental / Rational thinking / Intellectual understanding
Acceptance / Seeing life for what it truly is
Willingness / Willing to participate in life and contribute
Courage / Personal Power / Taking responsibility for yourself
Anger / Pride / Blaming others
Fear / Anxiety / Blaming self
Depression / Blaming self
Guilt / Shame / Blaming self
Low, bad-feeling energy

It is also important to understand that the higher the level or frequency of an emotion, the more in alignment you are with your True Self and the Great Universal Intelligence. So this is what your Inner Compass is telling you. Your Inner Compass lets you know that the higher you are on the emotional scale in terms of how you regard life, other people, and yourself, the better it feels. Because you are more and more in harmony with the Great Universal Intelligence that created you and this entire Universe.

So to sum it up, the higher the level of energy or frequency, the better it feels. In general, people who are higher on the emotional scale are happier in their daily lives. In other words, their experience of life is happier than the experience of people who are lower on the emotional scale. In addition, the energy of the higher frequency emotions is much more powerful than the energy of the lower frequency emotions. So when your energy is high, you not only feel better and more expansive, you are more powerful. And your ability to help and influence other people in positive ways increases because you are in alignment with the Great Universal Intelligence which is All-Powerful Infinite Energy. While when you are experiencing less good-feeling emotions, your energy is low because you are out of alignment, and so you don't enjoy life as much – and your ability to be of benefit to yourself, your family, and the world around you decreases.

Thus it turns out that following your Inner Compass and feeling good is also the very best way you can be of service to other people! So take good care of yourself if you want to be a positive influence in the world.

You are the only one who has access to your Inner Compass

Here's another thing that's important to understand: You are the only one who has access to your Inner Compass. Now why is this so? Well, it goes back to the Nature of Reality, the nature of this thing called Life. If you look at the Nature of Reality carefully, you will see that you are the only one who is inside of you. You are the only one who can think your thoughts and feel what you are feeling. Nobody else can get inside of you and know what it feels like to be you. Nobody else wakes up in your body in the morning and goes around inside you all day long, so nobody else in the whole wide Universe can possibly know what it's like to be you. Other people can guess; they can speculate, they can ask questions, they can assume. But they can't *know*. Only you can know what it feels like to be you because you are the only one inside of you. This is why no one else has access to, or contact with, your Inner Compass. Because the Inner Compass is inside you. It's a "feeling" mechanism that is working inside of you.

So the Inner Compass is based on the reality that no one else can "feel" for you. This is important to understand and consider. So just mull over this for a little while and notice that no one else can "feel" for you. It's like breathing – no one else can breathe for you. Or eat your food for you, either.

So remember this when you are in doubt about the Inner Compass. Remember that no one else can know what Life "feels" like to you, or what things feel like to you. Only you can feel and know this.

Thus, no one else can know what gives you a sense of pleasure, or a sense of ease and flow in your Life. Only you can. You are the only one who can feel and know this. You are also the only one who knows what doesn't feel good to you. Only you can know this because you are the only one inside of you. Only you can "feel" for you.

So please beware – when someone else tells you they know what you are feeling, or what's best for you! Because how can they know this? All they can do is assume that they can "feel" what you are feeling – but they cannot possibly "know" with any certainty what you really feel. This is just not possible! So how can they claim they really know what's best for you? Which is why I say – take care when someone claims to know what's best for you.

When we understand this, we can also see that it works the other way too. We don't have access to anyone else's Inner Compass either. And this tells us that no matter how close we are to another person, and no matter how much we love this person, we still don't have access to their Inner Compass and to what it feels like to be them, simply because we are not inside them. We don't have access to their "feelings" – we don't have access to how Life "feels" to them. Therefore, we don't have access to their Inner Compass either. So again – beware when you think you know what's best for someone else! How can you possibly know since you're not inside them?

No universal standard – no one size fits all

Because each person is different, in a different situation, at a different time in their life and evolution, there is no universal standard – no "one size fits all" – as to what's best for every single person on the planet, at any given moment.

Just consider this: The information that each individual is receiving from their Inner Compass is based on a multitude of constantly changing factors and information, which is based on who this person is and where he or she is in their life journey and evolution. As well as where the person is on the Emotional Scale (see page 30). So what feels good to one person may not feel good to another. It all depends on who you are and where you are, in terms of your life and your development. This is also why each person has his or her own Inner Compass – because we're all different. Each one of us is unique.

When we understand that each person is unique and that we are all different in various ways, we can also understand why there's no "one size fits all". Each one of us is a unique creation of the Great Universal Intelligence that created and is animating everything that is. It's kind of like our fingerprints. Each one of us has a unique fingerprint. No two fingerprints are identical, which is why the police and the authorities use our fingerprints to identify us. No one else has your fingerprint and no one else has mine. The Inner Compass is like that too. You have your own Inner Compass and internal guidance system and I have mine. You have your own specific connection (Inner Compass) to the Great Universal Intelligence, which is based on who you are, where you are, where you are going, and everything else about you. And I have mine. Your Inner Compass only works for you and mine only works for me. And since your Inner Compass is inside you, you're the only one who has access to it. No one else can get inside you and have access to your Inner Compass. The same goes for me.

This also explains why some people prefer the quiet life in the countryside, while others love the hustle and bustle of New York, Paris or London. Is one better than the other? Or what about relationships? Some people are into open relationships, while others prefer monogamy and having only one partner for their whole life. Some people love working late, while others love getting home to the kids early. Some people want lots of kids, while others prefer not to have children at all. Some like to spend as much time as possible out in the wild, while others would never dream of doing something like that. Some like to meditate, others like to dance, while some people are always glued to Facebook and Twitter on their smartphones… and so it goes.

This is why it's so important not to compare yourself to anyone else – because no "one size fits all". Comparing yourself to other people will only get you into trouble because you are uniquely you. You are not someone else – you do not walk in anyone else's shoes – you walk in your shoes. Comparing yourself to anyone else will only confuse you and lead you away from your own truth and your Inner Compass.

When we understand all this, we also understand why the idea that there's one universal standard, or one right answer that will work perfectly for all people, in all cultures, in all countries, at all times, and for all age groups, is just plain screwy. Quite simply, because it's just not possible.

We are all on a learning curve

When you start playing around with the Inner Compass, it's also good to understand that the Inner Compass is only about NOW – about the present moment and how you are feeling in the present moment. So it's important to understand that whatever you discover you are feeling right now might change tomorrow or even in an hour from now. Because life is a fluid, ever-changing flow of energy and events.

In this connection, it also helps to understand that we are all on a learning curve. And by this I mean, we are all evolving – you, me and everyone else. So our needs, wants, dreams, desires, hopes – all of it – keep on evolving and changing too.

This is why the signals from the Inner Compass are also constantly changing because these signals are constantly adjusting to this fluid reality and evolution. Which explains why something which once felt good, might not feel so good now – because you changed or evolved. Or vice versa – something which once didn't feel so good, might feel better now. Again, because you changed and everything else probably changed too. So yes, because everything changes, including you – what is best for you in this now-moment is continuously in the process of changing too.

When we understand this, we understand that this means that there's no fixed, perfect point with one fixed, perfect solution that always remains true for you, me, or for anyone else. There is no static, right solution for all time. Everything is in flux and flow because everything keeps changing and evolving.

So the more you are able to "flow" with the flux and flow of Life, the easier you will find it is to enjoy Life – wherever you are. And this is what the Inner Compass is all about. When you listen to it and are open to the signals from the Great Universal Intelligence, it gets easier and easier to learn and adjust, and readjust and adjust again, to whatever is going on in and around you. And then you will discover that you are, quite simply, feeling better and better every day in every way!

Your Inner Compass never says "should"

Even though other people (our parents, society, etc.) might try to tell us what we "should" say, do, or feel, the Inner Compass never says "should". All the Inner Compass tells you is whether or not something feels good – honestly and without any explanations. So when you hear a voice inside you telling you that even if something doesn't feel good, you "should" do this or that anyway, you can be sure that voice is not your Inner Compass. That voice is probably your mother's voice, or your partner's voice, or your child's voice, or some well-meaning friend's voice... But the voice is definitely not your Inner Compass! Because the Inner Compass never says "should". There are no "shoulds" in feelings. Feelings are very straightforward – they are what they are. Feelings either feel comfortable or uncomfortable. It's as simple as that.

And everyone knows this! Everyone knows when something feels good. Everyone knows the difference between feeling joy and feeling frustration. Everyone knows the difference between feeling love and feeling anger. We can all feel the difference in these feelings. We all know what feels comfortable and what feels uncomfortable. This is not difficult for any of us to discern!

It's also important to know that when you hear the "should" voices of other people (either internally or externally) – whoever these people are, and however well-meaning they may be, you can be sure you are listening to information that is not relevant for you. Because the truth is – as I said before – no one else can get inside of you and have access to how it feels to be you. It's just not possible. And anyone who tries to tell you otherwise is confused – no matter how well-meaning that person may be.

So what this all means is that when someone, be it your father, your girlfriend, your sister, your child, your neighbor, gives you advice or tells you how to set your hair, brush your teeth, bring up your children, manage your partner, or just in general how to live your life – you are wise if you run as fast as you can for the nearest exit! Because nobody else can possibly know what's best for you – ever. Ever! And this is because – as I keep saying over and over again – you are the only one who's inside you and who knows what it's like to be you. You are the only person who has access to your Inner Compass. You are the only one who knows what things feel like to you. You are the only one who knows what feels best for you. It's simply not possible for another person to know this, because nobody else can get inside of you and walk in your shoes.

That's why – truly – the acid test for the Wise Ones is they never tell other people how to live their lives. They might be able to talk about basic principles and the law of cause and effect (in other words, that everything has consequences), but they never ever say they know what feels best for another person. Instead, the sign of a Wise person is when he or she says – only you know what's best for you... so you do what you like!

What about "intuition" or "the voice within"?

A woman came to me and was confused about listening to what she called her "intuition" or "following the voice within". She told me this story: "I lived in Copenhagen and I heard a voice within telling me it was time to move from Copenhagen to London. The thought of it felt terrible but I thought it was my intuition or the voice within giving me guidance, so I moved. It turned out to be a disaster. I regretted it bitterly."

This story brings up a common misunderstanding. There are many different thought streams that we can plug into – many different ideas and impulses – but not every thought stream or impulse is giving you information that is appropriate or life-enhancing for you. So how can you know? How can you judge when you get an idea or an impulse if this is good advice or guidance for you? There is only one way – by listening to your Inner Compass. Because your Inner Compass will immediately let you know if the thought or impulse feels good or not. In other words, by means of your emotions, your Inner Compass will let you know if the impulse is in alignment with who you really are or not. So all you have to ask yourself is – does this thought or impulse give me a sense of comfort or discomfort? A feeling of ease and flow or a sense of anxiety? And there you have your answer.

If this woman had known about the Inner Compass and understood the way it works, she wouldn't have moved because the idea of moving from Copenhagen to London gave her an immediate sense of discomfort…

What does the Inner Compass say?

Job offer
I get a great job offer and everyone I know says it's perfect. *But what does the Inner Compass say?* When I think about taking the job, I feel discomfort. Saying yes to the job somehow doesn't feel right. So I follow my Inner Compass and two weeks later something even better turns up!

Job offer – version 2
I get a great job offer and everyone I know says it's perfect. *But what does the Inner Compass say?* When I think about taking the job, I feel discomfort. Saying yes to the job somehow doesn't feel right. But I disregard the Inner Compass and take the job. From the minute I arrive at the new workplace, I get this sinking feeling inside. It turns out

that my new boss is a real psychopath…

Marriage crisis
My marriage is on the rocks. Should I get divorced or should I stay? I'm really in doubt about this and keep weighing the pros and cons of either solution. But no matter how much I think about it, either option doesn't feel good. Suddenly a new idea pops into my head – move out and get your own place so you can be on your own for a while and sort yourself out. *What does my Inner Compass say?* The new idea gives me an immediate feeling of ease and flow, so I decide to do that.

So should I always do what feels good?

When we talk about the Inner Compass, and noticing what feels good, and then doing it – some people naturally ask, "Does that mean I should always do what feels good to me? What about doing stuff that feels good in the moment – like drinking or self-medicating or overeating or indulging in other types of unhealthy behavior that feel good in the moment? What about that?"

This is a very valid question, so let's take a look at these types of activities. First of all, it's important to understand and notice in situations like this that sometimes an activity that feels good (like drinking or overeating) is simply an attempt to soothe the discomfort that has arisen from years of not listening to and following our Inner Compass. So because we have neglected the Inner Compass most of our lives (and many of us have), and instead have been people pleasers, or people who are afraid of doing what feels right for us because we're afraid of criticism and the disapproval of others – then it makes sense that we've accumulated a lot of internal discomfort. (See page 41 about what happens when we don't follow the Inner Compass.) When we understand this, we can also see that, at times, what "feels" good in the moment is not so much the Inner Compass speaking to us as an attempt to soothe the discomfort that's built up over the years from NOT listening to the Inner Compass!

So yes, this is where things can get tricky for many of us. And this is where we really have to notice and be sensitive to what's going on inside us.

Another way of answering this question is to be aware that if you drink to forget or soothe your pain, it might feel good in the moment, but tomorrow you'll wake up with a hangover. And if you continue to drink to soothe your discomfort, it will have long-term, destructive consequences for your health, life, employment and relationships. While if you follow your Inner Compass, you will continue to feel good the next day and the next.

Approval feels better than disapproval

Here's another point of confusion. Since we've been programmed to seek the love and approval of others (be people-pleasers) and not follow our Inner Compass from an early age, many people will go to great lengths to avoid disapproval because this "feels better" in the short term than following your Inner Compass, which might make people criticize you or disapprove of you! So we sacrifice our own alignment and integrity for the temporary approval of others. But unfortunately, the accumulation of discomfort that comes from not following our Inner Compass over the course of many years is far greater than the temporary relief we feel, in the short term, by avoiding the disapproval of others. Understanding this and noticing this in various situations and relationships is something that you can only learn over time as you begin working with the Inner Compass. So don't beat yourself up if you disregard your Inner Compass and go for approval in the short term – but begin noticing when this happens and notice the consequences it has on your life.

I believe that this approval-seeking behavior probably stems from our deep-seated animal instinct, that has told us for generations that exclusion from the flock could mean extinction. In other words, our historical roots go way back in time and the collective consciousness has been tribal-based for many, many generations. So much so that even today, many of us still often unconsciously feel that the disapproval of others could mean exclusion from the group (family, tribe) and may even threaten our survival. So when feeling this kind of anxiety, it's important to remind ourselves that society has evolved and that we in the West are privileged enough to live in democratic societies, which protect the rights of each individual to be who they are and to live the lives they choose (unless of course the individual is interfering with the rights of another person to live the life he or she chooses). For more about this, see the section on democracy on page 95.

What happens when you don't listen to your Inner Compass

Your Inner Compass is constantly sending you signals, but what happens when you don't listen to the signals and act accordingly? Well, the signals don't go away, they simply get louder and more powerful. So when you ignore your Inner Compass, it tries harder and harder to get your attention. This means that what started out as maybe a vague feeling of mild discomfort will become a stronger feeling of discomfort. If you still don't heed the signal and understand the information it is giving you but continue to move away from what's best for you, the signal from your Inner Compass will get even stronger. So the unease and discomfort become more and more pronounced. More and more powerful. When this happens, people start to feel really negative emotions such as nervousness, or anxiety, or fear, or depression, or irritation and anger. In other words, the feelings get stronger.

This is where many people begin to look for ways to cope with their feelings of discomfort. Since we don't understand the real cause of our discomfort, or know what to do about it, we begin to develop various coping strategies to numb the pain of these uncomfortable emotions. It could be, for example, that we overeat, or over exercise, or turn to drink or drugs, or pill-taking to ease the discomfort. Some people try to cope by losing themselves in work (and become workaholics), or in food (and develop eating disorders), or through shopping, gambling, sexing, or whatever. If this continues, this may also be where addictions really kick in. All of these strategies are attempts to soothe ourselves from the discomfort we are feeling. To soothe the uneasiness and anxiety we are feeling about ourselves and our lives. A discomfort and uneasiness that arises from not listening to the Inner Compass, and from being out of alignment with the Great Universal Intelligence. A discomfort that arises because we are not living in harmony with who we really are.

Then, if we continue to neglect the signals from our Inner Compass and continue to move away from being in alignment with who we really are – the next thing that happens is we start to get physical indicators of this lack of alignment. Symptoms such as headaches, backaches, stomach aches, muscular tension, etc. start to appear. All of these symptoms are indicators that we are not allowing and moving with the natural flow of energy in our lives. Indicators that something is out of whack in our energy systems. At this stage of unease (dis-ease), the symptoms are usually not chronic and tend to move around – in other words, they come and go in relation to how much we move back and forth or in and out of alignment.

Then finally, if we continue to disregard the signals from our Inner Compass, the signals will get even more powerful and may finally manifest as so-called "chronic" or "serious" illness. In this light, it is interesting to understand that so-called serious illness can be understood to be a signal that we are out of alignment with the Great Universal Intelligence and who we really are, a sign that the energy is not flowing harmoniously in our system. As anyone who has studied the mind-body connection knows, our bodies tend to manifest and out-picture (reflect) what is going on inside us emotionally. So it makes perfect sense that when we disregard the signals coming from our Inner Compass, it will show up in various bodily symptoms that indicate a lack of alignment with the flow of Life.

This also tells us that no matter what our present physical and emotional condition may be, coming home to ourselves, and going within and listening to our Inner Compass, and aligning with the Great Universal Intelligence can, and will, have a profound healing effect on our physical and mental health and well-being.

Negative emotion is your friend

When we understand that negative emotions are signals from our Inner Compass that we are out of alignment with our True Selves and the Great Universal Intelligence, we can see that negative emotions are actually a good thing. Because negative emotion is a signal from the Inner Compass telling us that we are off the beam and out of alignment with what is best for each of us. So instead of being afraid of negative emotions and feeling bad about feeling negative emotion, it is actually more helpful to remind yourself that your emotions are simply indicators, they are simply the Inner Compass' way of letting you know whether you are thinking and behaving in ways that are in harmony with the Great Universal Intelligence and who you really are – or if you are off course. The stronger the negative emotion, the stronger the indicator that you're off course.

Negative emotions are a little like putting your hand on a hot stove. Ouch! It burns! When something like that happens, you don't get mad at your hand for letting you know that you had better move your hand away from the hot stove if you don't want it to get burned off! You don't say to your hand, this shouldn't burn! No, instead you listen to the message your burning hand is giving you and you move your hand away! So negative emotions are the same thing. They are messages from within, which are trying to guide you in a direction that is more in harmony with your innermost being, with your True Self and the Great Universal Intelligence. The only real question here is – are you listening? Or are you keeping your hand on that hot stove?

When we understand this mechanism, we can also understand what a fantastic asset the Inner Compass is when it comes to living a happy life. Because your Inner Compass is always guiding you in the direction of true alignment, which translates into joy and happiness.

Yoga, mindfulness, meditation, positive thinking and the Inner Compass

Here's something else that's interesting to notice when we are talking about the strategies we employ to soothe the discomfort we feel when we don't follow our Inner Compass. Could it be that working with many of our self-help techniques such as yoga, mindfulness, meditation and even positive thinking may sometimes be – at least partially – attempts by many of us to soothe the pain and discomfort we are feeling when we aren't listening to our Inner Compass? Could it be that? Could it be that we may be turning, to some degree, to these very powerful and wonderful practices in an attempt to soothe the discomfort that comes from not following the Inner Compass?

But even if the answer to this question is "yes", please don't misunderstand me when I say this. I am not saying that these techniques, in and of themselves, are not extremely helpful and beneficial. Of course they are! And I, for one, am a person who has written many books about the benefits of all these techniques. But what I am trying to say here is – if stress, or overwork, or any other type of discomfort, has led you to yoga or meditation or mindfulness, it could also be a good idea to ask yourself why you are feeling this stress and discomfort to begin with. Are you feeling this discomfort because you are not listening to your Inner Compass? Are you stressed out because you are afraid to say "no" and set healthy limits for yourself (either at the workplace or in your family) because you're afraid that people will disapprove of you? If that's the case, then in addition to working with these excellent techniques, perhaps it's time to find and follow your Inner Compass as well!

When did the first "no" arise?

Here's another good awareness technique when it comes to understanding and using your Inner Compass. When you have an area, or areas, in your life where you are having so-called "big" or "serious" issues or difficulties today – it can be very enlightening and clarifying to look back at the way things developed in this area of your life. Because when you do, you will probably discover – if you take the time to slow things down a bit – that the first time an inner "no" arose to this situation or person was a long, long time ago. In other words, the first time you felt discomfort, or a sense of unease arose within you (a signal from your Inner Compass), was way before the situation became really problematic for you.

So give it a try. Try slowing things down in an area that's troubling you and see if you don't find that the discomfort of today began to make itself felt a long time ago. And you will probably see that it did. The only problem was, you didn't listen or take seriously the messages that were coming to you from within. Which is to say, you didn't notice, you didn't hear the signal – you didn't listen to your Inner Compass. Just think about it. Take, for example, a relationship that has become very problematic for you. When you look at the situation today, you will most certainly discover that there were signs or indicators that you were somehow off track with yourself in terms of this relationship long before things actually became really difficult.

But you weren't listening to your Inner Compass, you weren't paying attention to the discomfort you were feeling in the early subtle stages. But if you think back, you will discover the discomfort was there a long time ago. But because of the way you were brought up (trained, indoctrinated, programmed), or because of your belief systems and your desire to please people and/or avoid conflict, you disregarded the information coming from within. You disregarded the discomfort. You disregarded the signals coming from your Inner Compass.

But just because we disregard discomfort doesn't mean it will go away. Because if the discomfort is a signal from within that we are not in alignment with who we really are and with what's best for us, the discomfort will only grow and continue to grow as long as our behavior is not honoring the voice within us.

So again, I suggest paying closer attention to the feelings that arise in you that are coming from within. These feelings are the signals from your Inner Compass, which are telling you in every moment, in every situation, what is going on with you.

Your Inner Compass and your thoughts about yourself

The Inner Compass is not just giving you feedback about your relationship to other people and the world, it is also giving you feedback about your own thoughts about yourself. Just think about it. When you have negative thoughts about yourself such as "I'm not good enough", or "There's something wrong with me", or "I'll never be able to figure it out", or "It's all my fault" – all these various types of self-criticism and negative thinking make you feel an immediate sense of discomfort. Now isn't that interesting? But if we consider this in light of the Emotional Scale on page 30 which shows the different levels of energy, we can see that the feelings of discomfort are actually the Inner Compass letting us know that such negative, low frequency thoughts about ourselves are out of alignment with what the Great Universal Intelligence knows to be the truth about us. So the result is –

when you entertain negative, self-critical thoughts like this, it means you are out of alignment with who you really are and this, of course, brings a great sense of discomfort.

Likewise, when you shift your focus to softer, kinder, more moderate thoughts about yourself like "I'm doing the best I can", or "I'll figure things out", or "I'm sure it will work out okay", or "There were a lot of factors involved in this situation, so it can't be all my fault", or "Everyone is on a learning curve, including me" – you feel an immediate sense of relief. So again, your Inner Compass is letting you know that these more positive (higher frequency) thoughts are more in harmony with who you really are and with what the Great Universal Intelligence knows about you.

It's interesting to notice that self-critical thoughts are almost invariably very categorical – a kind of black and white thinking. In other words, the thoughts are not nuanced in any way, they are very either/or. They often translate into the childish belief that goes something like this "Either I'm perfect or I'm a complete idiot/failure". Which really has nothing to do with reality. In reality, no one is so-called "perfect" (whatever that means) and we all have our strengths and weaknesses. This is why categorical thoughts like "perfect" versus "failure" feel so uncomfortable. Because reality is always much more nuanced – reality is the middle ground, which is always flowing, changing, and evolving – just like you and I are. Self-condemnation and self-criticism, on the other hand, are a very negative focus and almost always based on unrealistic expectations to, and assessments of, ourselves and life in general. (For more about psychological maturity versus categorical, black and white thinking, see my book *Sane Self Talk – Cultivating the Voice of Sanity Within*.)

The above is one more good reason to listen to the signals from your Inner Compass – they will always let you know when you're getting off track – even when it comes to your own thinking about yourself!

Life activities: Is it "Survival", your "Passion" or just "In Between Stuff"?

Here's another interesting way to look at what's going on in your life. To do this, we can divide the activities in our lives into 3 different groups or categories as follows:

Survival	In Between Stuff	Your Passion
Work (a job) to:	All the stuff you	Things you are
Pay the rent	"could" do or feel	passionate about.
Feed your kids	you "should" do	Things that you
Survive		feel inspired to
		do.

So let's start with "Survival". Almost everyone I know has stuff they absolutely must do to survive, pay the rent, and feed their kids. And by this I mean stuff like going to work at a job that you might not love but feel you can do because you have to do it to pay the rent and feed your family.

Then there's what I call "Your Passion". Many of us have things we're really passionate about, but which we often can't make a living doing. Like being an artist, or surfing all day long, or running, or becoming a healer, or a dancer, or developing a new invention or technology. There are, of course, some of us who reach a point in our lives where we can actually make enough money to survive (and even live comfortably) by doing the things we love. When that happens, well, hallelujah indeed!

Using the three categories is another way in which you can use your Inner Compass to help you get a little more clarity in your life. Start by dividing the activities in your life into the three categories. Then plug into your Inner Compass and look at the three categories and see what happens. If you do this slowly, you will notice that you feel a sense of comfort, ease and flow when you are focused on activities that fall under the "Passion" category or under the "Survival" category. Why under the Survival category? Because survival is basic, it's the basic instinct in all living creatures. You (and your family) have to survive in order to be able to do anything at all in this life! So obviously, survival feels good!

But what about all the rest of the stuff in our lives? And this is where what I call the "In Between Stuff" comes into the picture. It's here I've noticed (especially from counseling so many people over the years) that many people are wasting a lot of their energy (and their lives) by using way too much time on the "in between stuff". And by this I mean, spending time on the stuff that feels pretty okay or just so-so, but which doesn't feel great like passion and which isn't necessary for survival.

If you look around, you will discover that so many people (and maybe even you) are running around doing all kinds of stuff that feels pretty okay and which they can do, but which, if they really listened to their Inner Compass, they would not do. Because when you really notice how the things in the "in between" category feel – well, they don't feel all that good – and they definitely don't feel great. The things in the "in between" category are just in between. Or we could say they are bearable or doable, but they don't make your heart sing. So what kinds of activities am I talking about? I'm talking about stuff like going to stupid parties when you don't really feel like going, or going out with people you don't really feel all that comfortable with. Or going to a movie or watching something on TV with your boyfriend/girlfriend/partner when you'd rather be reading a book or doing something else. Or... well, you get the idea. Whenever you're doing something you can do, but which you don't *really* want to do or have to do to survive. Most of these things are things you can do, things which are not that bad – it's not like you will die or anything if you do them. But the real question is – why would you want to waste your precious life force and precious life energy on stuff like this when there are other things, things which you really love and are passionate about, which are calling you? Why should you do stuff like this when there are other things, which are more in harmony with who you really are and what you really want? And again, when you listen to your Inner Compass, you will not be in doubt about any of this...

So how do we navigate wisely in all of this? How do we sort all this out? Well, to begin with just notice. Just notice what's going on and what you're doing. Just noticing how the various activities in your life fall into these three different categories will help you get in touch with your Inner Compass and how you really feel about things. And then, slowly, slowly, I suggest cutting down on the activities that fall into the middle category and focusing more and more on what you are passionate about.

What does the Inner Compass say?

Birthday party
My parents want to have a birthday party for my five-year old daughter. *But what does the Inner Compass say?* The thought gives me an immediate feeling of discomfort. But I'm afraid my parents will be upset if I say no, so I give in and agree. On the day of the birthday party, I feel really lousy and my daughter ends up getting sick. The next day I have a serious migraine and have to stay home from work. It takes me several days to recuperate from not following my Inner Compass.

Launching a new project
I've finished a big project that I've been working on for a long time and am now ready to launch it. But for some reason, every time I think about launching the new

initiative, I feel a real sense of discomfort. I can't explain to myself why because everything seems ready to go, but I decide to follow my Inner Compass and wait and let it go for a while. While letting the project be and doing other stuff, I suddenly get a brilliant new idea that will enhance the project hundredfold! Thank God, I listened to my Inner Compass and waited!

Something's wrong with me

I'm going through a challenging time and I get the thought, "Something's wrong with me." *But what does the Inner Compass say* to this thought? Believing this thought gives me an immediate sense of great discomfort. Then I try out the thought, "I'm an evolving human being and I have my challenges just like everyone else. That doesn't mean there's something wrong with me." When I think like this, I feel a lot better.

PART TWO:

Dealing with the fear of disapproval and other challenges

The fear of disapproval and other challenges

Since the fear of disapproval and trying to please other people are among the main obstacles to following the Inner Compass for so many of us, let's take a closer look at these phenomena.

But before we start, let me say most emphatically that when I talk about being a "people pleaser", I am not saying you should not treat other people with respect. And I am not saying you should not support your friends and family in their endeavors. Nor am I saying you should not be a kind, compassionate human being.

What I am talking about is when we say or do things, which go against our own integrity (our Inner Compass), because we want to please someone else or because we are afraid of their disapproval. I am talking about situations and activities where we disregard our Inner Compass and go against the voice within us because we want to please someone else and avoid their criticism. It could be our partner, our parents, our children, our friends – the list of possible people we believe we can displease is endless!

So why are we so afraid of displeasing other people? Why is it so important for us to get other people's approval? And why is it so important to other people that we do what they want us to do rather than what feels right to us? Why do they care so much – and perhaps even get upset when we say "no" to their requests or do something other than what they think we "should" do or want us to do? These are some of the conundrums I consider here in Part Two.

If I follow my Inner Compass, I'll make someone else unhappy

If we look a little closer, we'll see that the underlying fear that drives many people's attempts to get us to do what they want us to do (for example, by referring to some higher, so-called universal standard of "right" and "wrong") is the belief that if we do what feels right to us, and as a consequence don't do what they want us to do – then they will be unhappy. In other words, consciously or unconsciously they have linked their happiness and well-being to what we say and do (or don't say and do).

So if this is the issue – that if you or I follow our Inner Compass, we'll make someone else unhappy – the question is, can this be true? Can your choices or mine actually make another person unhappy?

In order to answer this question, we first have to take a step back and look at the nature of this thing called Life and how the mind works. When we look a little closer at what is going on we discover that each person's thinking, i.e. his or her thoughts and belief systems, is the cause of the way that person experiences Life and all the events in his or her life. So when an event or circumstance occurs and it harmonizes with what the person believes is "right", or "correct", or "good", or "appropriate", the person will "like", or "approve of" what is going on. And when an event or circumstance is out of harmony with what the person believes is "right, correct, good, or appropriate", this person will "dislike" or "disapprove" of the event or experience. So each person's reaction is based on their belief systems and thinking.

When we understand this, we can also see that because each person's experience is based on his or her beliefs, then each person is actually responsible for their own reactions and experience of Life. And this holds true, whether or not the person is aware of this mechanism. Because this is an impersonal, universal law – like the law of gravity – which holds true for everyone. And the law is: *Our thinking determines our experience.*

Since this is the law of Life, this also includes other people's reactions to what you and I say and do as well as their reactions to what you and I do not say or do not do. Their reactions are determined by their beliefs and their thinking. Not by what you or I actually say or do.

So it plays out like this: If a person thinks something you say or do is good – he or she will be happy, and if a person thinks something you say or do is less good – he or she will be less happy or even unhappy. So what does it have to do with you? The way another person reacts is completely beyond your control because you can't get inside another person's head and control the way another person thinks and reacts to anything.

Happiness is an inside job

When we understand this basic mechanism – that *our thinking determines our experience* – we also understand that happiness or unhappiness is not the result of outer circumstances, or events, or other people's choices and actions. But rather, happiness or unhappiness is the result of each individual's interpretation of what is going on. Thus we see that happiness or unhappiness is a purely subjective experience. (For more about this mechanism, see my book *Are You Happy Now? 10 Ways to Live a Happy Life.*)

This is why I always say happiness or unhappiness is an "inside job"! Because happiness or unhappiness all depend on how each person views and interprets the situations and circumstances he or she is living with and in.

This is the mechanism of mind: *Our thinking determines our experience.*

This is what determines your experience and my experience.

Things happen and then we each react according to our belief systems.

Things happen and we each react based on our background, upbringing, beliefs, and practiced ways of thinking and reacting.

So your happiness depends on your thinking.

And it's the same for your partner, your child, your parents, and your friends. Their thinking determines their experience. This is why happiness is an "inside" job – for everyone. There is no exception to this rule.

So what does this have to do with following our Inner Compass?

A lot.

Because many people are afraid that if they follow their Inner Compass, they will make the people in their lives unhappy. They mistakenly think or fear that their choices and behavior will displease others and be the cause of another person's displeasure or unhappiness. It could be their partner, their parents, their children, their friends. Again, the list of possible people we believe our words and actions might displease is endless! But it all comes down to the fear that if you or I do what feels best to us – it might make someone else unhappy.

But now that we understand the mechanism of mind – that each person's thinking and belief systems are what determine their experience – we can see that our choices cannot actually make another person unhappy. It's just not possible.

Different people react in different ways to the exact same situation

Let's look at how the exact same situation can elicit very different reactions from people, depending on how they look at the situation. Here are some concrete examples:

- *Two people get divorced:* Now what does this mean? The reality is a divorce is when two people who once lived together now go their separate ways. That's a divorce. But getting divorced can, and does, mean different things to different people. For one person, a divorce can feel like a tragedy, like the end of the world, so this person may be deeply depressed. For another person, a divorce is a celebration, a liberation, because now this person is finally free from having to deal with a relationship that wasn't working, so this person is happy, joyful. In both cases, the event was the same – two people who were together are no longer together. But because they had very different interpretations of the event, they also had very different experiences of the same event.

- *Your boss asks you to head a task force to deal with a challenging situation at your workplace:* Now what does this mean? The reality is that this is a work assignment. But again, getting an assignment like this can, and does, mean different things to different people. For one person, the assignment will seem overwhelming and the person will experience a lot of stress. For another person, the assignment will feel like a great honor and challenge, and the person will experience renewed energy and joy at work. In both cases, the event was the same – a work assignment. But because they had very different interpretations of the event, they also had very different experiences of the same event.

- *Your children are grown-up and move away from home:* Now what does this mean? The reality is children who once lived at home now no longer live at home. They aren't there anymore. But this again can, and does, mean different things to different people. So again, it depends. One person will experience their children moving away from home as a great loss and feel a sense of emptiness in their life. So for many, this can be a time of real crisis and soul searching. While others may enjoy their newfound freedom and having more time to focus on the things they never found time for when the children lived at home. But again, the event was the same – the children are no longer living with their parents. But because they had very different interpretations of the event, they also had very different experiences of the same event.

In all the examples above, there is an event – something happens – and then, as we have seen, different people have different ideas about what these events mean for them and their lives. And it is always our interpretations of events that determine our experience and how we get to live. So if you think divorce is terrible, that's what you experience. If you think divorce is a true liberation, then that's your experience. And the same goes for the new assignment at work. If you think it's more than you can handle, you'll experience stress, and if you are delighted at being given the challenge, you'll experience renewed energy. And so on... The important point to understand here is that in, and of, themselves, the various events have no meaning. They are just the things that happen in life. But we give them meaning by the way we interpret them. And this is true of everything that is happening in our lives. Everything.

The same holds true when you decide to follow your Inner Compass and someone gets upset. Let's say spending some time on your own this weekend feels good to you, but your partner gets upset because he, or she, had other plans for the two of you. Is this the only way your partner could react to your decision? Probably not. Just think about it. If 10 different people in 10 different relationships tell their 10 different partners they want some alone time this weekend, would each one of these 10 partners react in exactly the same way? No, of course not. Maybe some would get upset, but others wouldn't. Some might even be happy to have some time on their own too! But in every case, the reaction of each person depends on their belief systems and their beliefs about relationships, the world, themselves.

So when we understand the nature of this thing called Life, and understand that *our thinking determines our experience*, we also understand that the idea that you, or I, could possibly be responsible for another person's happiness, or unhappiness, is a flawed premise. It is a flawed premise because it has nothing to do with reality. Because the reality is, it is completely impossible to get inside another person's head and think for that person. Which means we cannot possibly be responsible for the way another person thinks, or for the way that person experiences Life.

But unfortunately, most people do not yet understand this basic mechanism. They do not yet understand that the experience of each individual person is completely – 100% – determined by that person's thoughts and belief systems.

And because most people do not yet understand the basic principle that a person's thinking determines his or her experience, most people continue to mistakenly believe that the happiness of other people must in some way depend on what they say or do. Moreover, they also believe the reverse is true, too – that their own happiness depends on what other people say and do.

Unfortunately, this misunderstanding can make it very difficult, if not impossible, for many of us to listen to the signals we are getting from our Inner Compass. Because – God forbid – what if the Inner Compass guides you in the direction of something your partner, or parents, or children don't like, or disapprove of!

So now you can see that this basic misunderstanding about who is responsible for each person's happiness is the reason why your parents, and mine, trained us to please them. This is also the reason why we train our own children to please us. Because we mistakenly believe that other people are somehow the cause of what we are experiencing. Thus, we believe that other people are responsible for the way we feel. We believe that what other people do makes us feel the way we feel – and therefore, they are responsible for our happiness.

And we believe the reverse, too. We believe that we are responsible for the way other people feel and react too – and therefore, somehow responsible for their happiness!

But this, as we can see, is not true.

So when you find yourself falling into the trap of believing you are responsible for someone else's happiness (and I promise you, you most probably will, because we all do!) – remind yourself of the universal law. Remind yourself that there is this thing called "reality" (the events and circumstances that are happening in our lives) and then there is our thinking and inter-pretation of these events. And that it's our interpretation of these events and circumstances that determines our experience – not what anyone else is saying or doing! (For more about this mechanism see my books *Are You Happy Now? 10 Ways to Live a Happy Life, The Awakening Human Being – A Guide to the Power of Mind* and *Sane Self Talk – Cultivating the Voice of Sanity Within*.)

But I know my partner will be upset!

Oh – but you say – I know if I do this or that my partner will be upset. And yes, it's true you *do* know your partner will be upset. You *do* know how your partner will react because you know what your partner's belief systems are. So yes, it's true, you do know your partner will be upset!

You know, for example, if you say to your husband I'm going away for the weekend with my girlfriends to Paris or I'm going to a silent meditation retreat for the next 10 days, he'll be upset if he's the kind of man who expects you to always be around and do all the things he wants you to do. But what does that have to do with you? All this tells us is what kind of a guy he is. All this tells us is what his belief systems are. It really has nothing to do with you. Because he could just as well respond differently and say, "How wonderful, sweetheart, I hope you have a great time." Or he could say, "That's great, I really need some alone time, too, so I'm happy you're going away." Or he could say, "Good for you, I was planning on going fishing with my buddies anyway…" Or he could say, "Do what you like!" So there's just no end to how people can react to whatever you say or do.

And it works the other way too. If you're expecting your partner to act in a certain way so that you can be happy – well, then you're the one who is giving your power away and making other people (who you can't control) responsible for your happiness. It's kind of like taking the people you love hostage! And that never works out well!

So how can we sort all this out? The Inner Compass is the only way! When we know and understand that each one of us has an Inner Compass, and we understand that happiness is an "inside" job, it becomes easy to take responsibility for the only thing we can control – and that is our own choices and the ways in which we respond to what is going on in and around us.

Take your power back!

So the belief that I am responsible for your happiness, or that you are responsible for my happiness, is probably one of the most disempowering beliefs in the whole wide Universe! Because it means you and I are giving our power away and making ourselves victims of other people and outer circumstances, which you and I cannot control. The same goes when someone else is trying to make you responsible for their happiness because then that person is giving his or her power away to you and making himself, or herself, a victim of outer circumstances (you), which they cannot control!

So if I believe my happiness depends on you, I am giving my power over my own life away to you! And if you believe that your happiness depends on what I say or do, you are giving your power over your own life away too. Because this faulty belief says you're not responsible for you and I'm not responsible for me! In addition, it implies that you don't have the intelligence and the resources to figure out what's best for you! And it says the same about me if I give my power away to you or anyone else.

All of this is the exact opposite of the Inner Compass principle, which in essence is all about self-empowerment. Because the Inner Compass principle says that you have an internal guidance system that is directly connected to the Great Universal Intelligence and that it is always giving you clear infor-mation as to what is in harmony with you. Which means that you can figure things out for yourself and that you can take responsibility for your own life and your own happiness!

And this is Good News indeed!

So take your power back and start noticing when you are disregarding your Inner Compass and the signals that are coming from within you instead of trying to figure out what you believe you need to say or do to make other people happy – and then STOP doing it!

Instead remind yourself of the principles of this Universe (reread the start of this section), and remind yourself of the fact that happiness is an "inside job", and that each human being is responsible for their own happiness, and for learning to be in alignment with the Great Universal Intelligence and what feels best and most appropriate for them – wherever they are in this thing called Life.

Then remind yourself that everyone else has an Inner Compass and a direct connection to the Great Universal Intelligence... just like you do.

And then listen, once again, to your Inner Compass!

People who are out of alignment want you to fix them

Here's another aspect as to why it can be so important to another person (my partner, mother, son, daughter, friend) that I do what he or she wants me to do.

When we look closely at what's really going on, we will almost always discover that when a person is very dependent on another person's behavior for their own happiness, it's a dead giveaway that this person is, in some way, unhappy or unfulfilled in their own life. For some reason, this person has lost contact with their own Inner Compass and is out of alignment with who they really are. So the person is not really in flow and living the joyous, fulfilling life he or she was born to live. When this happens, a person like this may look to outside forces, or other people, to fix them, fulfill them, and make them happy.

This confusion arises for many of us because we don't understand that we have our own Inner Compass and our own direct connection to the Great Universal Intelligence, which is always guiding us towards the happiness and fulfillment we seek. So when a person depends on someone else to fix them or make them happy, this person obviously doesn't realize this. Moreover, he or she doesn't realize that he or she is feeling discomfort because they are out of alignment with what harmonizes with their true nature. Instead, the person often mistakenly thinks that they are feeling discomfort because of what another person is saying or doing. Then they wrongly think if only they can get their partner (or children or family) to do what they want them to do – then they will feel good again. But their discomfort has nothing to do with other people – it's all about being out of alignment with who they really are!

So you can see the whole thing is backwards and screwy!

Because the opposite is true. When people are in alignment with who they really are and are living happy, fulfilled lives, they are usually too busy having a good time to care so much about what other people are doing, or are not doing, with their lives. Someone who is listening to his or her Inner Compass and making good choices is a person who is in flow. A person who is in flow is joyous, and enthusiastic, and having a good time – and someone like this doesn't make other people responsible for their happiness. They know they are responsible for their own happiness and are enjoying their journey, every step of the way.

Arbitrary standards of behavior

When people try to pressure you into doing what they want you to do (because they, consciously or unconsciously, believe that getting you to do what they want will make them feel better), they usually don't do this by saying directly, "My happiness is dependent on you! If you don't do what I want, I'll be miserable."

(Although some might actually say this outright!) Most people will instead often try to get you to do what they want by appealing to some higher standard of behavior, some arbitrary standard of "right" and "wrong", to justify their request. They will either say, or imply, that, "This is simply how we do things" in our family, in our country, in the Western world, if we're good Christians, if we're good Jews, if we're good Muslims, etc., etc. What is implied here is that there is some higher standard involved that we have either forgotten, overlooked, or don't quite have the intelligence as individuals to figure out for ourselves, which is more important than any silly ideas we might have as to what feels best to us.

And this has been the case for most of us. From early childhood, most of us have been trained/manipulated by our parents, teachers, friends and others (all with good intentions, of course), who have tried to control our behavior by appealing to some arbitrary universal standards of right and wrong. Standards, which many of us have never quite figured out or understood. But whether or not we understood them, from childhood on, it has been implied that there are some higher standards, which we, in our imperfection, need to follow. And since we're not bright enough to figure this out for ourselves, we need to be controlled and corralled into place by having other people (who seemingly know more than we do) point out to us the inappropriateness of our behavior. And they do this by telling us that our behavior is either improper, indecent, immoral, or somehow unacceptable because it doesn't match the standard they're going by (whatever that happens to be). People who use tactics like this may include our mothers, fathers, sisters, brothers, partners, other family members, our children, cousins, neighbors, people at work – you name it. There are people like this everywhere you turn. But in every case, it is usually someone who is not good at simply asking for they want – for example by saying – "I would prefer if you'd..." or "I'd really like to you..."

and who is then able to respect your answer. Instead, non-assertive people like this try to manipulate you into doing what they want by appealing to some higher, arbitrary standard of perfection that they say you are not living up to.

Unfortunately for us, the consequence of all this is that if we, ourselves, actually do believe there really are some higher, arbitrary standards of right and wrong out there that are better able to determine what is right or wrong for us than we are, then we're easy targets for other people to manipulate... which also makes it difficult to look within, and find and follow the signals from our Inner Compass.

For more about arbitrary standards and how to avoid being manipulated by them, see my books *Are You Happy Now? 10 Ways to Live a Happy Life* and *Sane Self Talk – Cultivating the Voice of Sanity Within*.

What if my family doesn't like it?

So what if your Inner Compass tells you to do something that goes against the wishes of your family? What then? What do you do?

Give up your dream? Don't listen to your Inner Compass? Grit your teeth and get on with your family's plan for you and your life?

It's a good question isn't it? And this is where so many people get into trouble, even if they know in their heart of hearts what they want to do. It could be, for example, choosing a career track your family doesn't approve of, or being in a same sex relationship, or marrying someone of a different race or religion, or dropping out of school or going back to school, or changing jobs, or quitting your job or... the list of things you might want to do that your family might disapprove of is endless. (It all depends on your family and their belief systems!)

So what can you do?

If you don't want to give up your right to be you and follow your Inner Compass, this is where it's important to remind yourself of everything that's in this book about you being you, and you having a right to be you, and you having an Inner Compass that is always telling you what is best for you. And remind yourself that we are fortunate enough to be living in democratic societies, which protect the rights of the individual to live the life that he or she chooses. (For more about this, see the section on democracy on page 95.) So think upon these things over and over again until you are sure you understand the basic principles. Remind yourself that it's not your job to make other people happy, but that it is your job to follow your integrity and support everyone else in following theirs!

And then... once you've reminded yourself of all of this, it is also important to realize that this is where assertiveness training comes into the picture.

Why assertiveness training? Because if you're in a situation where other people disagree with you or your choices or projects, it's important to learn how to take care of yourself, set healthy boundaries, and say no when something doesn't feel right to you (to your Inner Compass). This is what being assertive is all about. Being assertive means that you can take care of yourself when other people interfere with your right to be you, and make the decisions which feel best to you. In fact, learning to be assertive actually makes it much easier for you to follow your Inner Compass because you know you can take care of yourself when you are guided to do something that the people around you might not approve of. Nothing helps reduce anxiety like assertiveness training!

In this connection, it's also important to understand that being assertive is something most of us have to learn to do, and then practice doing. Being assertive is not something we automatically know how to do. It doesn't happen overnight, even though most of us were naturally assertive when we were little kids. But unfortunately, we usually have had our natural assertiveness trampled out of us at an early age when our parents, and our surroundings, trained us to be people-pleasers and do what they wanted us to do, instead of following our own inner guidance.

Your assertive rights

When it comes to learning to be assertive, a good place to begin is to read and think about the list of assertive rights below that were mapped out by Manuel J. Smith in his classic assertiveness book *When I Say No, I Feel Guilty.*

Your assertive rights, i.e. your right to be you and live your life the way you choose, include all of the following:

"Assertive Rights

1 You have the right to judge your own behavior, thoughts, and emotions, and to take the responsibility for their initiation and consequences upon yourself.
2 You have the right to offer no reasons or excuses to justify your behavior.
3 You have the right to judge whether you are responsible for finding solutions to other people's problems.
4 You have the right to change your mind.
5 You have the right to make mistakes – and be responsible for them.
6 You have the right to say, 'I don't know.'
7 You have the right to be independent of the goodwill of others before coping with them.
8 You have the right to be illogical in making decisions.
9 You have the right to say, 'I don't understand.'
10 You have the right to say, 'I don't care.'

You have the right to say no, without feeling guilty. "

Once you start to understand these basic rights, the next challenge is how to actually integrate and apply this understanding when dealing with other people who are trying to persuade you, pressure you, or manipulate you into doing what they want you to do. So let's take a brief look at what to do.

The "sandwich technique"

A good basic technique to start with is the "sandwich technique", which is a positive, assertive way to respond to other people's demands. The sandwich technique is about responding to other people's requests or demands with sentences or statements, which are made up of two different parts.

In the first part of the sentence, you acknowledge to the other person that you have heard what he or she said. In the second part of the sentence, you give your response. In other words, you tell the person what you think, or feel, about his or her request or demand (i.e. how your Inner Compass is responding to the situation).

So when using the sandwich technique, a good assertive response (which is made up of these two parts) basically sounds like this:

- I hear what you're saying and I feel differently about the matter.
- I really respect your opinion and the way I see it is like this…
- Your friendship means so much to me and I'm going to have to decline your kind offer.
- I understand what you're saying and this is not something for me.
- Thank you for thinking of me and I have other plans for the weekend.
- I really appreciate you thinking of me and I have other plans for Saturday night.
- I can see this really means a lot to you and I'm going to have to say no.

- Yes, I can relate to what you're saying and from my point of view, it looks to me like...
- Thank you for thinking of me, I really appreciate your concern, and no thanks.

This is a skillful way to deal with whatever people are requesting, or demanding, because you begin by acknowledging that you hear the other person and that you understand what he or she is saying (and even appreciate their interest). Then after that, you come with your response, which is your no, or you setting limits and following your Inner Compass.

Here are some examples:

Example one: You get invited to a party this weekend. The signal from your Inner Compass is one of discomfort so you decide not to go. Here's your conversation with the host.

Host: "We're really counting on your coming to our party on Saturday."

Your response: "Thank you so much for thinking of me and I can't make it that evening."

Host: "But we're counting on your coming."

Your response: "I really appreciate your thinking of me and I can't come that evening."

If the person keeps on, you just keep repeating what you said. Sooner or later the other person will give up.

Example two: You get a new job offer. Your Inner Compass doesn't have a good feeling about this and you get the feeling there's something better in store for you.

Your friend/your mother: "I really think you should take that job, it's such a great opportunity for you."

Your response: "Yes, I can relate to what you're saying and it's simply not for me."

Your friend/your mother: "But can't you see what a great job opportunity this would be for you. It would be so good for your career."

Your response: "Thank you for your concern and this job is simply not for me."

Again, if the person keeps on, you just keep repeating what you said until the other person gives up.

When you learn to respond assertively to other people's requests in this way, it's good to remember the other person probably won't agree with you, and doesn't have to. Being assertive is not about winning arguments, convincing other people, or being right. Being assertive is about setting limits and taking good care of yourself. It's not about winning and losing. So be willing to hear and acknowledge the other person's point of view ("You could be right"), and then clearly state your own position ("and it's not for me").

Remember, it's your job to listen to your Inner Compass and take care of yourself in relation to what is going on. The other person is responsible for his or her feelings and opinions about the matter. Each person has a right to his/her feelings and opinions. You don't have to justify yourself, offer explanations, or find excuses for your choices. (You might want to explain, but the important point to remember is that you don't have to. You have the right to be you and offer no explanation for your choices.)

So to summarize, here are the main points to keep in mind:

- Acknowledge that you hear the other person.
- Then deliver your response.
- Use the word "and" when connecting the two parts of the sentence because the word "and" is inclusive.
- Don't expect the other person to agree with you.
- Don't be afraid to repeat yourself, kindly but firmly.
- You are responsible for your feelings and your decision about the matter.
- The other person is responsible for his/her feelings about the matter.

Here are some more good ways to acknowledge the other person's point of view while maintaining your own rights, position, and point of view. You can say things like:

- I understand you feel that way and in my experience, I find that...
- You could be right and I prefer to do it this way...
- I can understand your point of view and I would rather not...
- I really appreciate your input in this matter and I still...
- I appreciate your thinking of me and the answer is no.

And finally, learning to say no, set limits, and be assertive like this takes practice. It's not something one learns in a day or two, it really does take practice. In the beginning, it can help to rehearse situations in your head before and after they occur, especially if you've been in situations where you didn't respond assertively in a good way. Try going through these situations in your head and visualizing how you would like to tackle these situations the next time they come up. The more you practice in your head, the more you will discover that you can actually do this when situations like these arise in your daily life.

Here's another tip for beginners. When you find yourself in a situation where someone catches you off guard with a request and you're not sure what your Inner Compass is saying or how to respond – ask for time to consider the matter.

Asking for time

If you're new to listening to your Inner Compass and unsure how you feel about something, it can be a good idea to ask for time when somebody asks you to commit to something.

So you can say: "Thank you for asking. Let me think about it. I'll get back to you." Or, "I'll have to check my calendar. I'll get back to you." So even though the Inner Compass is always giving you guidance right now, many of us have to gradually learn to listen to it and follow it. Asking for time will help you in two ways:

1) It gives you time to get quiet and notice what your Inner Compass is really telling you about this person, event, situation, invitation, possibility – if there's a feeling of comfort or discomfort or if there's another option, which feels better to you that you can suggest instead.

2) It gives you time to practice an assertive response if your answer is no and you know that the other person might get upset or try to press you into saying yes.

So let's go back to one of the examples above and see how asking for time works:

Example one: You get invited to a party. You're not sure how you feel about this yet.

Host: "We're really counting on your coming to our party on Saturday."

Your response: "I really appreciate your thinking of me; let me look at my calendar and I'll get back to you tomorrow."

Host: "But we're counting on your coming."

Your response: "I really appreciate you're thinking of me and I'll get back to you tomorrow."

If the person keeps on, you just keep repeating what you said.

By postponing your response in this way, you give yourself time to listen to your Inner Compass and then to plan how to deal with the situation assertively when you call back and respond.

Working with assertiveness

If you find it challenging to be assertive, in addition to the above, I suggest you get a good book on assertiveness training. You can also find more about being assertive in Chapter 3 of my book *Are You Happy Now? 10 Ways to Live a Happy Life,* and in my book *Sane Self Talk – Cultivating the Voice of Sanity Within.* Then begin practicing these assertiveness techniques until you learn that there are skillful ways of communicating with other people so they understand where your boundaries are. Being assertive means you can learn to tell people you have a different opinion or plan than they do in a good, firm, and yet appreciative way. When you learn to do this, when you learn the art of being assertive, you will discover three things. Firstly, to your great and everlasting delight, you will discover that when you are assertive most people respect you even more than they did before. Secondly, you will also notice that nobody dies when you defy the will of your family or partner or children or colleagues. And thirdly, you will understand that you don't need the approval of other people all the time to live a happy life. (Yes, believe it or not, it's true. You weren't put on earth to please your family and other people even if that's what they'd like you to believe.)

But, as I said, learning to be assertive is not something you can accomplish overnight. You will, however, discover that as you become more and more stable in listening to your Inner Compass and being assertive, it will become easier and easier for you to interact in constructive and positive ways with everyone you meet. Why? Because you will have a deep inner knowing that no matter what anyone says to you – you can figure things for yourself because you have an Inner Compass and you know how to be assertive and engage in constructive and positive dialogue with people, whether or not they agree with you and your thoughts, decisions, choices.

When people continue to make you "wrong"

Unfortunately, even when we learn to be assertive in a good way, some people will continue to judge our behavior or choices as "wrong" and start telling us how to live our life. If this happens – especially when it happens repeatedly – it can be helpful to set healthy boundaries with responses like this:

- I know you mean well and when you say that you're

making my life choices wrong. That's not a constructive way for us to talk. If we are going to continue having a good relationship, please talk respectfully about my choices and my way of doing things.

- I know you mean well and when you say that you're telling me how to live my life. This is not a constructive way for us to be together, so I'd appreciate it if you would mind your own business. If I want your input or advice about my lifestyle, I will be sure to ask you.

And finally, if this kind of disrespectful and/or offensive behavior continues, you might want to consider staying away from this person as much as possible or even dropping the relationship altogether.

(For more about healthy boundaries, see my books *Are You Happy Now? 10 Ways to Live a Happy Life* and *Sane Self Talk – Cultivating the Voice of Sanity Within.*)

Minding your own business

In the above, we're talking about dealing with people who are "minding your business" – i.e. people who are giving you advice when you haven't asked for their advice, or telling you what to do, or trying to pressure you into doing something that doesn't feels right to you (to your Inner Compass). But obviously, when it comes to minding one's own business, it works both ways. So it's equally important that you and I mind our own business as well and refrain from giving other people advice unless they ask for it.

There are two main reasons why minding your own business is the wisest course of action.

First of all, when we understand the Inner Compass mechanism, we understand that everyone has an Inner Compass and that everyone is having their own unique experience of Life. When we understand this, we also realize that we can't possibly know what's going on inside another human being. It's just not possible. We don't have access to that information. This means that you and I cannot possibly know what's best for another human being because we don't have contact with their Inner Compass. So it's not possible to judge what's best for someone else – we simply can't know this. Moreover, it's disrespectful of the other person's intelligence and ability to figure out life for him or herself.

The second reason why it's so important to mind your own business is this: When we try to mind someone else's business, we are using a lot of our own precious mental energy thinking about, worrying about, and/or trying (at least mentally) to control someone else. When we do this, we lose contact with ourselves. We lose contact with our Inner Compass and our own internal guidance system because we're so occupied with what the other person is, or other people are, doing. So that's the other big backside of minding someone else's business – you lose contact with yourself! You become disconnected from yourself. And this leads to all kinds of problems such as feeling unfulfilled and unsatisfied with your own life.

So when we understand this, minding your own business is obviously the wisest way to live. And it's always such a relief too because it means staying in your own space and taking good care of yourself. Which frees up so much mental energy, and allows you to tune into your own Inner Compass, and find out what really feels good to you. When you do this, you find you are able to make better, wiser choices for yourself. Choices, which are based on an inner knowing – and in that way, you find you are able to live more happily, and you become a positive influence in the world around you.

So mind your own business! Set everyone free in your mind – for your sake and for theirs! Don't interfere with others unless they specifically ask for your help. And trust that everyone has the resources and intelligence to figure things out for themselves, just like you do! (For more, see the chapter "Mind Your Own

Business" in my book *Are You Happy Now? 10 Ways to Live a Happy Life.*)

The Inner Compass and children

Since everyone has an Inner Compass, this means that children do too. But what does this mean in practice for parents and teachers? How do we respect the fact that each child has an Inner Compass without allowing children to become "spoiled brats" or "petty tyrants"? There is a lot of confusion about this, so let's take a look at what's going on.

When we have children, it's the parents' job to provide a safe platform for the child to grow up and develop. Providing a safe platform includes providing a safe home with food, clothing, education, medical care, emotional support, etc. All of this is the parents' job and parents do this best by creating a home where there are clear, basic guidelines, or ground rules, as to how we, human beings, can live together in peace and harmony while respecting each individual's right to be who he or she is. And this includes our children.

The basic ground rules in the home are pretty much like the rules of traffic. Red lights mean stop, green lights mean go. You drive on the right in this country (in some countries, you drive on the left). The speed limit is… on the highway and the speed limit is… in town. We all know about the rules of traffic and we all know that if we drive through a red light, or drive faster than the speed limit, we can get a ticket or be arrested. It's not a question of whether we like these rules or not, these are just the ground rules we humans have agreed upon and set up to facilitate the way people can live and move around together in the best possible way without crashing into each other. So if you get stopped by the police because you were speeding, they don't ask you how this makes you feel or if you like the law. They're not interested and don't care – all they know is you broke the law (the ground rules). And that has consequences.

The same goes for good parenting and the basic ground rules for peaceful living in a family. And this is where many parents get confused. Kids don't get a say in making the basic ground rules – that's the parents' job. And kids don't have to like the ground rules – they just have to know they exist and understand that there are consequences if they do not follow or break the ground rules.

This has nothing to do with allowing, or not allowing, children to feel their emotions. And this has nothing to do with respecting the fact that every child has an Inner Compass. Breaking the basic ground rules and experiencing the consequences is one thing. Feeling your emotions is another thing. So when a child breaks a ground rule, it has consequences whether or not the child likes it. Parents are often confused about this and want their children to "like" or "feel good" about following the ground rules and about the consequences of breaking the rules. But this is impossible. It's impossible to expect children to always "like" or "feel good" about following the ground rules. And this is where parents get confused. Children can dislike the ground rules at times and that's quite okay. The psychologically mature parent understands this and is able to say, "I know you don't feel like washing your hands before dinner, but that's the way we do things here in this house. When you're grown-up and have your own home, you can decide to do things differently, but as long as you live here, this is the way we do things in this house."

Parents are not respecting their children's right to be who they are and feel their feelings and the signals from their Inner Compass when they try to prevent their children from feeling what they are feeling. So it's important to distinguish between what the ground rules are and how children feel about following them. These are two different things. So if a child dislikes a ground rule, that is his or her right and privilege as a human being because that's how the child feels. But this has nothing to do with following the ground rules. A child can dislike a ground rule all he or she wants, but the child has to follow it or there are consequences. It's as simple as that.

So the clear message from the parent to the child should be: "This is the ground rule about this matter in this family, whether or not you like it and regardless of how you feel about it. If you break the ground rule, the consequences are..."

The confusion arises when the parent wants to control how the child feels about the ground rules and the various situations. Because then the message from the parent to the child is – *you shouldn't be "feeling" what you are feeling. You should feel the way I want you to feel. You should be happy and like something because I want you to.*

This is emotional abuse from the parent's side because the parent is telling the child that he or she doesn't have the right to feel what they are feeling. The parent is basically telling the child what he or she "should" feel. This is disrespectful behavior from the parent's side.

Healthy, respectful behavior from the parent's side says – "The ground rules in this house are that we wash our hands before dinner and we brush our teeth before we go to bed at night." The child can like this or not, but these are the rules – just like traffic regulations. And it's the parent's job to set up the guidelines and make the ground rules for the home – not the children's. A home where children are growing up is not a democracy. It's the job of the mother and father to decide on the basic ground rules for living harmoniously together – but that's it!

This is not the same as saying that parents get to choose the child's pathway in life. In other words, it's not the parents' job to choose what subjects the child likes best in school, who the child likes to play with, what sports the child likes best, who the child wants to be friends with, what kind of books the child best likes to read, and how the child feels about a multitude of things and situations. Each child has an Inner Compass that is naturally guiding him or her in the direction of what feels best for them.

And obviously, as children get older, the wise parents respect their children's intelligence and ability to make these choices for themselves. (The wise parent will try to explain to their children that everything has consequences, but that is not the same as trying to control a child's choices and preferences.) This also means that when children become teenagers, it's not the parents' job to decide who they are going to date, what career path they are attracted to, who he or she might want to marry, etc. All of this is the job of the young adult. And as children mature and become teenagers and young adults, the wise parents will encourage them to find and follow their Inner Compass when it comes to figuring out what's best for them and finding their pathway in life.

The lure of glamour, fame and success

The fear of disapproval and feeling responsible for the way other people feel are not the only reasons why following the Inner Compass can be so difficult for so many of us. There are other reasons why people get sidetracked from their internal guidance system. In a world where there is so much glamour and where we are all constantly online, comparing ourselves to other people all the time, it can be easy to get sidetracked and lose touch with our own integrity. This can happen when we become enamored by the glamour of things like:

- Fame
- Success
- Money
- Popularity
- Recognition
- Looking good (appearance)
- Sex
- Possessions
- etc.

The lure of things like this can be very difficult to withstand and should not be underestimated. I have worked with people (young and old) who have not listened to their Inner Compass for one or several of the reasons above. The result has always been the same. They lost touch with their integrity and got so off course in their life that they usually ended up in some kind of crisis situation.

When working with people like this, I have found that they usually discover – when looking more deeply at what is going on in their lives – that they wanted success, or fame, or money, or popularity so badly that they disregarded their integrity and the signals from their Inner Compass. As a result, they ended up in all kinds of difficulties and, in the end, were having trouble living with themselves.

So again, to live a happy, fulfilling life, it is so important to understand that you have an Inner Compass which is providing you with all the information you need to navigate a healthy and happy pathway through the challenges you are meeting in your daily life. And that the consequences of constantly comparing yourself to what other people are saying and doing at the cost of disregarding the signals from your Inner Compass can be extremely distressing, to say the least!

Self-referral or other-referral?

Another way of looking at and understanding this mechanism is to understand the difference between "self-referral" and "other-referral".

When you have self-referral, your point of reference is within you. Your reference point is your Inner Compass, which is your direct link to the Great Universal Intelligence. Some people might call this connection, your connection to your True Self, which *is* the Great Universal Intelligence! So when you have self-referral, your decision-making process is based on your Inner Compass, which is your connection to your True Self and the Great

Universal Intelligence.

Unfortunately, for many people, their point of reference is other people and the beliefs, opinions, and ever-changing likes and dislikes of other people. And this is what I mean by "other-referral". Other-referral is when you look to other people for guidance in your decision-making process instead of looking within and following your own Inner Compass and your own connection to the Great Universal Intelligence. When there is other-referral, your responses are based on how you believe, or assume, other people will react to you and what you are saying and doing. And since you may want to avoid the disapproval of others at all costs, you might also disregard the signals you are receiving from your Inner Compass. This is what happens when our need for approval overrides our ability to have self-referral. And as we have seen, the emotional and physical toll of this type of behavior can be quite damaging over the long term.

This is also why spiritual practice such as meditation and spiritual study can be so helpful because it strengthens our ability to turn within, follow our Inner Compass, and come into alignment with our True Selves and the Great Universal Intelligence, which created all of us and this entire Universe.

The difference between "self-referral" and "other-referral"

Looking for guidance

Self-referral	Other-referral
Looks within, to the Inner Compass	Looks without, to others

Looking for cues as to how to behave & what to say

Looks within, to the Inner Compass	Looks without, to others

Wondering how to respond to challenges & various situations

Looks within, to the Inner Compass   Looks without, to
                                            others

Unsure of what to eat, wear, post on Facebook, where to go on
holiday, etc.

Looks within, to the Inner Compass   Looks without, to
                                            others

Wondering how to respond to a political or social issue

Looks within, to the Inner Compass   Looks without, to
                                            others

The power of two or more in alignment

We live in a Universe governed by law and one of the basic laws or principles of the Universe is "like attracts like". (For more about these laws, see my books *The Awakening Human Being – A Guide to the Power of Mind* and *The Road to Power – Fast Food for the Soul*.)

This universal law – that like attract like – governs everything in our lives including the kind of people we attract into our lives. The interesting thing here is that the better your energy is, and the more you listen to your Inner Compass and are in alignment with the Great Universal Intelligence, the more you will attract people into your life who also have good energy and who are also in alignment with the Great Universal Intelligence. So this is a really interesting phenomenon to understand and notice. Because when two or more people, who are in alignment with the Great Universal Intelligence, get together and join forces, it's a really powerful experience. Really powerful, really productive – and lots of fun too! The combined energy, flow, creativity and joy of two or more people who are in alignment with the Great Universal Intelligence is truly a powerhouse and an amazing force for Good in the world. Because the thing is, when people like this come together, it's more than a one plus one plus one relationship going on. In reality, there's an exponential factor involved here, which makes the energy and influence of two or more people with high energy coming together so powerful. You will find this phenomenon referred to as the "Master Mind" group or the "Master Mind" concept by various teachers. (I discuss this in my book *The Road to Power – Fast Food for the Soul* in the chapter entitled "The Power of Friends".)

This phenomenon applies to all types of relationships – whether we're talking about business partners, friends, couples, colleagues, sports teams, business teams, artistic groups, social and political movements, etc. There have been many examples of this throughout human history such as the Founding Fathers of the United States whose powerful new ideas were to change the course of human history. Others good examples include Peter and Eileen Caddy, the founders of the Findhorn Community in Scotland, the Inklings – the writers' group at Oxford that included JRR Tolkien and CS Lewis, Jesus Christ and his disciples, Buddha and his disciples, or artistic groups or partnerships like the Beatles, or Henry Miller and Anais Nin. Not to mention the worldwide 12 Step groups and the powerful dynamic that arises in these groups when it comes to healing addictions that have been otherwise impossible to deal with.

What does the Inner Compass say?

Trouble with my boss
My boss is always late for meetings and it's really annoying to me and the other employees, but I don't say anything because he's my boss. The more I think about it, the more inner stress and discomfort I experience. I find I'm almost starting to hate the guy. Then one day I get so pissed off at

my boss that I decide to speak up. *But what does the Inner Compass say?* The moment I think about asking my boss to come to our meetings on time and kindly respect me and the other employees, I feel much better, even if it might mean losing my job.

Wedding
My good friend was about to get married for the second time. A few weeks before the wedding, he met another woman and he really fell for her. His gut feeling told him to cancel the wedding because thinking about the coming wedding gave him a real sense of discomfort. But he didn't follow his Inner Compass because he felt he couldn't disappoint all the people involved and because he was afraid of breaking his wife-to-be's heart. So he went through with the wedding and got married. But after the wedding, in fact right from the start, things didn't go so well. My friend really, really tried to feel good and be excited about his new wife... but it didn't work. And then... after a while he started having an affair with the other woman. He just couldn't help himself. And as you can guess, he finally ended up having to tell his new wife how he really felt and they got divorced. After a while, he married the woman he loved all along and the two have been very happy together for many years.

Momentum and learning to use the Inner Compass

So you have now read most of this book and have begun trying to be mindful of your Inner Compass and notice how you actually feel about what's going on in your life. But try as you may, you are also discovering that this is not always easy to do. Now why is this so? Why can something, so seemingly simple as noticing the signals from your Inner Compass, at times be so difficult to do?

The answer to this important question is that when it comes to learning to use your Inner Compass, your old mental habits and practiced behavior (such as worrying about what other people may be thinking about you) can be very difficult to change because these old mental habits have gained a lot of momentum over time. And by momentum I mean the speed or the amount of energy that is behind these practiced ways of thinking. It is important to understand that because we have been practicing these flawed ways of thinking and behaving since childhood, the momentum behind these thought patterns, and this type of behavior, has increased over the years. Which can make this behavior very powerful today – and difficult to change.

It can help to understand this if you think about it or visualize it like this: Your habitual ways of thinking and behaving are like the Titanic – which is a very huge ship. And by this I mean your mental habits, or thought patterns and conditioned responses, are like a really big ship that is sailing in a certain direction. Moreover, this ship is going very fast because it has a lot of power and so it has gained a lot of momentum. What is more, your ship is moving in the direction you've been practicing for years and years.

Then one day you discover the Inner Compass and you decide you want to change your course. You want to change the direction you're sailing in. You want to change your mental habits and stop focusing on what other people may be thinking about you and start focusing, more consistently, on your Inner Compass and what's going on within you. In short, you want to change the direction of your thinking and sail in the opposite direction. So you decide to give it a try but you discover it's not so easy to do because your old thought patterns and behavior (conditioned responses) just seem to kick in all the time.

This might make you feel really discouraged and you might even think it's not possible for you to change the direction of your thought. This is when it's really important to remind yourself of what's really going on here. To remind yourself that the problem is *momentum*. And here the image of the Titanic can help you. Because it's like you suddenly want to turn this gigantic ship, the Titanic (or your habitual thought patterns), around and sail in the opposite direction. And this simply can't be done. Everyone knows that you can't suddenly turn a really big ship like the Titanic around and sail in the opposite direction all at once. It's just not possible.

But we all also know that you *can* turn a really big ship like the Titanic around, little by little. In other words, even though you can't turn a big ship around on a dime, you can turn it and change the direction the ship is going in, little by little. And that's exactly how it works when it comes to changing the way you think, and your conditioned responses, and practiced behavior. You can't turn your thinking around all at once, just like that. It's just not possible because you have so much momentum going in the direction of your old thought patterns. But with regular, persistent mental training – you can, little by little, day after day, practice new patterns of thought.

And this is where Mental Training comes in.

Mental Training

I call learning to change your habitual thought patterns – Mental Training. I call it Mental Training because changing the direction of your thoughts takes real diligence, discipline, and practice.

The reality is, Mental Training is just like any other kind of training and practice. You have to start small and keep at it for days, weeks, and even months, until you build up enough momentum in the new direction so you actually begin to change the direction of your thoughts. (For more about Mental Training, see my books *The Road to Power – Fast Food for the Soul*, *The Awakening Human Being – A Guide to the Power of Mind*, and *The Mental Laws*.)

Mental Training is like learning to play the piano or training to run a marathon. You don't just sit down and play like a concert pianist. Just like you don't just go out and run a marathon! To play like a concert pianist or run a marathon, you have to start small and build up your practice. When it comes to running, for example, first you must start running short distances and then you must practice running longer and longer distances. Everyone knows this. Everyone understands that you slowly have to build up your stamina and strength, and gradually increase the distance you can actually run – especially if you want to run a marathon. You can't just suddenly do it. But if you keep at it, if you keep running, then one day you may actually be able to run a marathon! But this doesn't happen overnight. On the contrary, it takes real practice and dedication – and it takes time. And the same goes for changing your mental habits; it takes real practice, discipline and dedication – and it takes time!

But it's certainly worth the effort – especially when it comes to the Inner Compass and you understand that the more often you are able to let go of worrying about what other people may be thinking and return to your Inner Compass, the easier it will become for you to actually go within and feel what is best for you!

Awareness is the key

So now that you understand the mechanism and how difficult it can be to change habitual patterns of thought and behavior, you can also understand there's no point in beating yourself up or calling yourself a "failure" because you can't immediately change the direction of your thinking and put all this new understanding into practice overnight.

Instead, it's a better idea to praise yourself for your growing awareness of the mechanism and principles. Praise yourself for your new understanding of the Inner Compass. Because without being aware of what's going on – it's impossible to change anything!

It's so important to understand and remember that: Awareness is the key!

Remind yourself over and over again that before you can make any real, substantial changes in your thinking, behavior, and life, you must understand the mechanism and principles involved. So first of all, a basic understanding and awareness of the whole Inner Compass principle is crucial before any change in your thinking and behavior can happen. Then realize that by understanding the Inner Compass principle and thinking about it, you are actually beginning the process of change.

So go back and read the beginning of this book again. Go back and review the basic principle of the Inner Compass again and again until you are quite sure you understand it. Then make the decision to do the Inner Compass exercise outlined on page 17 over and over again. Make the decision to try to focus on your Inner Compass during the course of your day. And then get to work and understand that to simply notice what you're doing during the course of your day is the best place to start. Try to focus on your Inner Compass and your feelings, and then simply notice where your thoughts are. When you discover you are worrying about what other people may be thinking or saying about you or the situation at hand, just shift your focus gently away from them again, and return back to yourself. Just gently return home to yourself, and go within, and listen to what your Inner Compass is telling you about whatever is going on.

Just notice what you are honestly feeling.

Notice what's going on inside you.

Notice if the situation gives you a feeling of comfort or discomfort. And be honest about what you discover. Don't try to censor your feelings because you think you "should" feel in a certain way and don't! You don't need to do anything, just notice and be aware!

Then pat yourself on the back and say – isn't it just great that

I'm waking up and have grown so much in self-awareness that I can actually see what's going on and honestly notice what I am feeling.

It's a process – a never-ending process

It's also important to remember that finding and following your Inner Compass is a never-ending process. Not only does it not happen all at once, it's a continual ongoing process of noticing and readjusting. Noticing and readjusting. And this will continue for the rest of your life! Because the Inner Compass is a minute by minute, hour by hour, thing – and it's all about just noticing what the Inner Compass is saying. Because the Inner Compass' response to Life is a fluid, ever-changing indicator that you slowly become more and more aware of. So it's a never-ending story, just like Life is. A constant process of growth and evolution.

When you understand this and get the hang of it, you can actually start enjoying yourself more and more because you know that wherever you go and whatever happens, you have an Inner Compass that is connected to the Great Universal Intelligence, and is always guiding you and giving you the information you need to make wiser and wiser choices! All you have to do is listen in!

So we're right back at the beginning again and the big question is: Are you listening to your Inner Compass now? And are you listening in now? Do you understand that your emotions are important and that they are always giving you clear and valuable information about what is best for you? And if the answer is yes – well, then, great glory and wonder! It means you are learning to take better care of yourself! It means you can be truer to, and more in alignment with, who you really are, which also means you can be a much greater force for Good in this world!

So hallelujah for the Inner Compass!

What does the Inner Compass say?

Trying hard to find a solution
I'm in a challenging situation and I keep trying and trying to find a solution to the problems I'm facing. But the more I think about it and the harder I try, the worse it feels. Suddenly I have a new thought: Maybe I should just give up and drop the whole thing for a while? *What does the Inner Compass say?* The moment I stop trying so hard to figure things out, I feel instant relief.

Should I quit my day job?
I really want to be a healer and do it full-time – and quit my day job. I'm also a single mother with two kids to support. *What does the Inner Compass say?* The thought of quitting my day job gives me a strong sense of discomfort – so I decide not to quit my job. But I still want to practice my healing arts, so I start using my free evenings to give healing sessions to friends and family. When I do this, I experience a strong sense of joy and exhilaration.

A sudden impulse
I am going to town to go shopping for jeans and shoes and I have my route and the shops I want to go to all planned in advance. Suddenly I get an impulse to go to that old café down by the harbor. But my mind says no, you don't really have time and it's out of the way. But the impulse is so strong and when I think about it, it feels so good. So I follow my Inner Compass and go there anyway. And guess what? While sitting in that old café enjoying a cup of coffee I meet the love of my life!

EPILOGUE:

The Inner Compass and human evolution

Democracy – the highest form of government

The understanding that each individual has their own connection to the Great Universal Intelligence is also the basis of our democratic way of life.

Democracy is a social system that is based on the right of each individual to be who he or she is. All democratic societies are based on the idea of respecting the individual's right to live life as he or she deems best – as long as the individual does not interfere with the rights of the next person to live his or her life as he or she feels is best. So you can see, this system of governance is based on the understanding that each individual is unique and has an idea of (and access to) what feels best for them. In other words, each person has an inner knowing or an "Inner Compass", which is, at all times, guiding that individual in the direction of what is best for them at any given moment in time.

The founders of the American Declaration of Independence understood this and so wisely wrote in 1776:

> We hold these truths to be self-evident, that all men are created equal, that they are endowed by their Creator with certain unalienable rights, that among these are life, liberty and the pursuit of happiness.

All the laws in our democratic societies are attempts to regulate the interactions between individuals based on this concept of freedom so that we each respect the rights of others while attempting to live our lives in the way we each deem best. And of course, this can, at times, be very difficult and challenging, and this is also why we live in societies that are law-based. All our laws are an attempt to regulate this interaction as fairly and justly as possible.

In short, you can say – in a democratic society, you have the right to stand on your head all day long, if that's what feels right to you, as long as you don't interfere with my right to stand on my head all day long, if that's what feels best to me. So this freedom goes both ways, allowing each of us to live as freely and fully as possible while respecting the rights of our neighbors to live their lives as freely and fully as they can, and as they deem best.

Unfortunately, in my work as a therapist and coach, I've discovered that even though we live in so-called "democratic" societies, many people in families and couple relationships don't respect the rights of their respective family members to live their lives as they think and feel is best. Instead they often try to shame, blame, manipulate, or coerce other family members into living life the way they believe is best for them. And this is not only extremely disrespectful, it is also the cause of much disharmony and abuse in many families and relationships. Sadly, this misguided behavior is caused by a fundamental lack of understanding that each individual is a unique creation and has an Inner Compass, which is always guiding them towards what feels best and most harmonious and joyful for them.

So the idea of consensus – as nice as it sounds in theory – cannot really work in families unless there is, first, a deep understanding and respect for the fact that each individual family member has a unique destiny path, which is based on the information they are receiving from the Great Universal Intelligence via their Inner Compass.

It is important to remember there is no "right" way – no "one size fits all" for every member of any family. Families like societies are multifaceted and constantly changing.

Consensus or flock mentality?
It's also interesting to note that from an early age, children in school are so influenced or guided (or misguided) by peer

pressure or the power of the group. The longing to be liked and accepted, the fear of being disliked, or criticized, or mocked, is so great in most that it takes an awful lot of courage for a child, or young person, to think, be, look, or act "differently". To stand out from the crowd or flock. And when you combine this with the fact that most children have not learned from their parents that they have a right to be who they are and to follow their Inner Compass, it's easy to understand how peer pressure can get ugly and turn into "mobbing" or bullying, with all the psychological and emotional damage that ensues.

When we go a little deeper, we discover that what's going on today with children is a logical consequence of what children have learned from their parents. Because the reality is, most parents are also terrified of being different, of not living up to what they perceive to be the "right" way of looking, acting, or living in their particular group – which might result in being criticized, judged, or God forbid, excluded, or ostracized from the flock (the tribe, the group, the family). So how can parents teach their children to be respectful of each individual's right to be who they are, and listen to their Inner Compass, if the parents themselves are too insecure or afraid to do this?

The basic problem here is the misunderstanding or ignorance of the basic principles I am writing about in this book, which include the basic principles of democracy. And because of this lack of understanding, parents do not act as if they know and understand that each person has a right to be who they are and that each person has an Inner Compass. So how can they teach this to their children if they do not understand and practice this in their own daily lives? So until we as adults understand the mechanism of the Inner Compass and all that it entails, we cannot expect the behavior of children at school to be different.

Being inclusive comes naturally when we understand that everyone is a unique creation and has their own direct link to the Great Universal Intelligence.

Fortunately for all of us, even if we are confused about these basic principles and terrified of displeasing others, we also know at some deeper level that this doesn't feel right. And this is because we all actually do have an Inner Compass! An Inner Compass that actually engenders a real sense of discomfort when we are out of alignment with who we really are. The other thing to remember is that everyone has a deep, natural urge within to be free. Yes, everyone wants to be free! Just think about it…

Everyone wants to be free!

This is a good thing to meditate on. No one ever fights to be a slave – have you noticed? Everyone wants to be free. Everyone, all around the world, regardless of age, sex, color, religion, nationality – we all want to be free. Even little kids want to be free! Yes, everyone does! No one wants their freedom interfered with or tampered with. Just think about it. No one wants their freedom blocked or hampered.

So we discover it's our natural, inborn nature to want to be free. We're just born like that. It's the way we are, it's how we're wired. Freedom is so important to us that we're willing to fight and die for it. No one ever fights to be a slave. So that's the way we all are – from the moment we are born. And we're all like that.

No one wants someone else telling them what to think, feel, do, or say. And yet, what do we humans do? We are constantly interfering with each other's freedom – all day long. From morning to evening with all our "you should do this" or "you should do that" stuff. It's completely crazy. And it goes completely against the grain of our innermost nature.

But please don't misunderstand me. I'm not saying we don't need some guidelines for healthy interactions between people. As I said above – that's what democracy is all about. But besides the basic laws that regulate our interactions with our fellow human beings, the idea that one person can possibly know what's best for another is completely absurd! Completely. Because it goes against reality. And the reality is – as I've said throughout this book – that no one can get inside another person's head and think and feel for them. No one can walk in another person's shoes. And because of this, no one can know what's best for you besides you!

So the idea that I could know what's best for you or that you could know what's best for me – or that you or I could possibly know what's best for someone else – is completely off the mark. Fortunately for us, our democratic society is based on an under-standing of this – which is why democracy is the highest and best form of human society, because it's based on the reality of how we really are. The reality that everyone wants to be free.

So when we understand this, we can also understand that one of the very best guidelines for living happily with our fellow human beings is this: Set other people free in your mind and *mind your own business! Mind your own Inner Compass instead!*

The Inner Compass and human evolution

And finally... when we understand the Inner Compass mechanism, we can also see that all human evolution and progress have occurred because someone was brave enough to follow their Inner Compass and walk new pathways despite the opinions of the majority. We call people who do this – visionaries and pioneers. But really, they are just people who are listening to and following their Inner Compass. They are the people who are strong enough, and have courage enough, to say, "Well yes, humanity may have been doing things like this for thousands of years, but I believe we can do things a little bit differently. So I think I am going to try this..." This is how all the great new discoveries, inventions and works of art have come about – whether it's a Galileo saying the earth moves around the sun, or a Bill Gates who revolutionized computers, or a Bob Dylan revolutionizing music and changing the course of a generation, or gay people standing up for their human rights, there have been, and still are today, countless people who are doing things differently and in new ways. People who are doing things in ways, which often turn out to be of great benefit to the rest of us. Fortunately for all of us, there have always been, throughout the course of history, people who have had such a strong sense of their Inner Compass that they have had the courage to walk new pathways.

And this is what all human evolution is about!

So if you are in doubt about listening to your Inner Compass when it tells you to tread new pathways, please remind yourself that this is what all human evolution is about. Then try to cultivate a little bit more of a sense of wonder or "beginner's mind" as you go about your day. And say to yourself, "I wonder where this will lead me? I don't know, but it feels good so I am going to give it a try. It will be exciting to see how this unfolds!"

Wouldn't this be a lovely way to live?

What did the Inner Compass say to Barbara Berger?

A life-changing meeting
During the Vietnam War, when I was 20 years old, my husband Steve and I were in Mexico City on the run from the US Army. Steve had been drafted and we were against the Vietnam War. We had been underground for 2 years and never told anyone what we were doing or running from. One day in 1966, when we were sitting on a park bench in the middle of Mexico City not knowing what to do next (we had only $150 dollars in our pocket), a man we didn't know came up to us. The man asked us if he could sketch our faces because he was an artist. We said yes. He sat down before us on the grass and started sketching. Suddenly he put down his pad and asked us what we were doing in Mexico City? For some reason, I had a strong

impulse to tell this stranger the truth, even though we had never told anyone before. And for some reason, it felt good. So I followed my Inner Compass and told this complete stranger everything about our situation. I told him that we were running away from the US because of the war, and that we were afraid and didn't know what to do. He immediately said not to worry – he said that he thought we were doing the right thing and that he would take care of us! Just like that. And he did! It turned out he was Ragnar Johansson, a famous Swedish painter, and he really did take Steve and me back to Sweden, changing the course of my life forever!

One Final Word: Everyone and everything responds to love

If you are still in doubt about the Inner Compass, just consider this. Everything and everyone responds to love. Everything and everyone responds to kindness. It's not something you have to learn. You don't go to school to learn that love feels good. It just does and you know this. It's not something mental or something you have to think about. You know love feels good. You just do.

Babies respond to love, have you noticed? They know what love feels like from the very first breath. They don't have to learn it. Babies don't need their mothers and fathers to explain to them that love feels good. They just respond to love because it feels good.

Actually everyone knows love feels good. We all do because it just does. And so does kindness. So you can ask yourself – how do we know – how do you and I know that love feels good? How?

Isn't that interesting?

Well, we just do.

We didn't have to learn that love feels good did we? Just like we don't have to learn that anger and fear feel bad. We just know this.

It's an inborn knowingness – an inbuilt mechanism, an inbuilt feeling awareness that we are all born with. We just know what feels good and what doesn't. And love and kindness feel good. And it's the same for everyone and for animals too. Just think how animals respond to love… they don't have language, they're not mental, but still they know what love feels like and they respond to it. Think about your dog or cat. Even plants respond to love as many gardeners know…

Which is why I can say with absolute certainty that you – and everyone else – has an Inner Compass. Because we all know what love and kindness feel like.

Acknowledgements

This book is uniquely my own teaching.

But no teacher stands alone.

Everything I teach and write about is based on what I have learned, and experimented with, and practiced, based on a lifetime of exploring this thing called Life. My teachings have been profoundly influenced, formed, and guided by the teachings of many amazing teachers and explorers in the field of consciousness including:

Abraham – through Esther & Jerry Hicks

David R. Hawkins

Byron Katie

Eckhart Tolle

Emma Curtis Hopkins

Emmet Fox

Ernest Holmes

Therapists such as Peter Levine, Pia Mellody and the 12 Step programs

Manuel J. Smith

& many other of the world's greatest teachings such as Buddhism, Advaita (non-dualism), the Bhagavad Gita, the New Thought movement.

My gratitude to these amazing human beings and teachings cannot be expressed in words.

In addition, this book is based on my many years of doing private sessions with people – and seeing what works and what doesn't work when it comes to helping people find their true inner power and move forward more joyfully in their lives.

And last but not least, many thanks to my editor, Tim Ray, for his invaluable assistance throughout the whole process of forming and delivering the powerful and important information about the Inner Compass contained in this book.

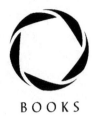

BOOKS

O-BOOKS

SPIRITUALITY

O is a symbol of the world, of oneness and unity; this eye represents knowledge and insight. We publish titles on general spirituality and living a spiritual life. We aim to inform and help you on your own journey in this life.

If you have enjoyed this book, why not tell other readers by posting a review on your preferred book site? Recent bestsellers from O-Books are:

Heart of Tantric Sex
Diana Richardson
Revealing Eastern secrets of deep love and intimacy to Western couples.
Paperback: 978-1-90381-637-0 ebook: 978-1-84694-637-0

Crystal Prescriptions
The A-Z guide to over 1,200 symptoms and their healing crystals
Judy Hall
The first in the popular series of five books, this handy little guide is packed as tight as a pill-bottle with crystal remedies for ailments.
Paperback: 978-1-90504-740-6 ebook: 978-1-84694-629-5

Take Me To Truth
Undoing the Ego
Nouk Sanchez, Tomas Vieira
The best-selling step-by-step book on shedding the Ego, using
the teachings of *A Course In Miracles*.
Paperback: 978-1-84694-050-7 ebook: 978-1-84694-654-7

The 7 Myths about Love...Actually!
The journey from your HEAD to the HEART of your SOUL
Mike George
Smashes all the myths about LOVE.
Paperback: 978-1-84694-288-4 ebook: 978-1-84694-682-0

The Holy Spirit's Interpretation of the New Testament
A course in Understanding and Acceptance
Regina Dawn Akers
Following on from the strength of *A Course In Miracles*, NTI
teaches us how to experience the love and oneness of God.
Paperback: 978-1-84694-085-9 ebook: 978-1-78099-083-5

The Message of A Course In Miracles
A translation of the text in plain language
Elizabeth A. Cronkhite
A translation of *A Course in Miracles* into plain, everyday
language for anyone seeking inner peace. The companion
volume, *Practicing A Course In Miracles*, offers practical lessons
and mentoring.
Paperback: 978-1-84694-319-5 ebook: 978-1-84694-642-4

Rising in Love
My Wild and Crazy Ride to Here and Now, with Amma, the
Hugging Saint
Ram Das Batchelder
Rising in Love conveys an author's extraordinary journey of

spiritual awakening with the Guru, Amma.
Paperback: 978-1-78279-687-9 ebook: 978-1-78279-686-2

Thinker's Guide to God
Peter Vardy
An introduction to key issues in the philosophy of religion.
Paperback: 978-1-90381-622-6

Your Simple Path
Find happiness in every step
Ian Tucker
A guide to helping us reconnect with what is really important in
our lives.
Paperback: 978-1-78279-349-6 ebook: 978-1-78279-348-9

365 Days of Wisdom
Daily Messages To Inspire You Through The Year
Dadi Janki
Daily messages which cool the mind, warm the heart and guide
you along your journey.
Paperback: 978-1-84694-863-3 ebook: 978-1-84694-864-0

Body of Wisdom
Women's Spiritual Power and How it Serves
Hilary Hart
Bringing together the dreams and experiences of women across
the world with today's most visionary spiritual teachers.
Paperback: 978-1-78099-696-7 ebook: 978-1-78099-695-0

Dying to Be Free
From Enforced Secrecy to Near Death to True Transformation
Hannah Robinson
After an unexpected accident and near-death experience,
Hannah Robinson found herself radically transforming her life,

while a remarkable new insight altered her relationship with
her father; a practising Catholic priest.
Paperback: 978-1-78535-254-6 ebook: 978-1-78535-255-3

The Ecology of the Soul
A Manual of Peace, Power and Personal Growth for Real People
in the Real World
Aidan Walker
Balance your own inner Ecology of the Soul to regain your
natural state of peace, power and wellbeing.
Paperback: 978-1-78279-850-7 ebook: 978-1-78279-849-1

Not I, Not other than I
The Life and Teachings of Russel Williams
Steve Taylor, Russel Williams
The miraculous life and inspiring teachings of one of the
World's greatest living Sages.
Paperback: 978-1-78279-729-6 ebook: 978-1-78279-728-9

On the Other Side of Love
A Woman's Unconventional Journey Towards Wisdom
Muriel Maufroy
When life has lost all meaning, what do you do?
Paperback: 978-1-78535-281-2 ebook: 978-1-78535-282-9

Practicing A Course In Miracles
A Translation of the Workbook in Plain Language and With
Mentoring Notes
Elizabeth A. Cronkhite
The practical second and third volumes of The Plain-Language
A Course In Miracles.
Paperback: 978-1-84694-403-1 ebook: 978-1-78099-072-9

Quantum Bliss
The Quantum Mechanics of Happiness, Abundance, and Health
George S. Mentz
Quantum Bliss is the breakthrough summary of success and spirituality secrets that customers have been waiting for.
Paperback: 978-1-78535-203-4 ebook: 978-1-78535-204-1

The Upside Down Mountain
Mags MacKean
A must-read for anyone weary of chasing success and happiness – one woman's inspirational journey swapping the uphill slog for the downhill slope.
Paperback: 978-1-78535-171-6 ebook: 978-1-78535-172-3

Your Personal Tuning Fork
The Endocrine System
Deborah Bates
Discover your body's health secret, the endocrine system, and 'twang' your way to sustainable health!
Paperback: 978-1-84694-503-8 ebook: 978-1-78099-697-4

Readers of ebooks can buy or view any of these bestsellers by clicking on the live link in the title. Most titles are published in paperback and as an ebook. Paperbacks are available in traditional bookshops. Both print and ebook formats are available online.

Find more titles and sign up to our readers' newsletter at http://www.johnhuntpublishing.com/mind-body-spirit

Follow us on Facebook at
https://www.facebook.com/OBooks/
and Twitter at https://twitter.com/obooks